BOUNDLESS
HEALING

Tulku Thondup

BOUNDLESS HEALING

MEDITATION EXERCISES TO ENLIGHTEN THE MIND AND HEAL THE BODY

SHAMBHALA · *Boston & London* · 2000

SHAMBHALA PUBLICATIONS, INC.
Horticultural Hall
300 Massachusetts Avenue
Boston, Massachusetts 02115
www.shambhala.com

9 8 7 6 5 4 3 2 1

First Edition

Printed in the United States of America

⊗ This edition is printed on acid-free paper that meets the
American National Standards Institute z39.48 Standard.

Distributed in the United States by Random House, Inc.,
and in Canada by Random House of Canada Ltd

Library of Congress Cataloging-in-Publication Data
Thondup, Tulku.
Boundless healing: meditation exercises to enlighten
the mind and heal the body/Tulku Thondup.
p.   cm.
Includes bibliographical references.
ISBN 1-57062-574-3
1. Meditation—Buddhism. 2. Mind and body. 3. Healing—
Religious aspects—Buddhism. I. Title.
BQ5612.T48 2000
294.3'4435—dc21
00-032202

CONTENTS

vii

Contents

FOREWORD

by Daniel Goleman

WE HAVE ALL HAD MOMENTS in our lives when we were so lost in a thing of beauty or in doing something, so completely absorbed that we were oblivious to nearby distractions or the passing of time. Those luminous moments are treasures, spontaneous leaps into another mode of being—one where day-to-day preoccupations or anxieties fall away, where we are somehow lifted out of our usual burdens.

Psychologists study that state under the name *flow*, a word that refers to the fluidity people experience in what they do at such moments. From the perspective of emotional well-being, flow states are peak experiences, moments when we are at our best, when our mind is at peace. They cannot be scheduled or programmed; they come to us as gifts.

The essence of that gift is a mind and heart at peace. With the flowering in recent years of scientific findings on the links between mind and body, there is growing proof (for those who need it) that entering such peak states bodes well for physical health. There is little question now that positive moods boost the immune system's resistance to germs and viruses and lower the risk of heart disease.

To be sure, the lotteries of life—genetics, stresses, and the like—all have their role in our susceptibilities. But one health risk factor we should be able to have direct control over is our state of mind.

Yet modern medicine—with its boggling arsenal of machines and pharmaceuticals—cannot tell us how to put ourselves into the inner states that seem to have positive health benefits. Happily, there are other systems for healing that have mapped that terrain well.

Here, Tulku Thondup offers a masterly synthesis of methods from the Tibetan tradition that he has found conducive to inner peace. He goes a step further than he did in *The Healing Power of Mind*, here detailing an extensive set of practices designed to cultivate peace of mind and facilitate physical well-being. These methods, based on classical Tibetan practices, allow us to share in a way to train the mind to tap into its own healing power.

As he points out, even as modern medicine continues to flourish, we in the West also have unprecedented access to ancient knowledge and means for healing the mind and body. Why not avail ourselves of both?

ACKNOWLEDGMENTS

I OFFER MY HEARTFELT GRATITUDE to the third Dodrupchen
Rinpoche and his nectarlike article "Turning Happiness and Suffering into the Path of Enlightenment"; to my enlightened teachers and
caring friends; to my loving parents and forebears; and to all who
shared their wisdom, inspiration, and stories for this endeavor. This
book would not even have been conceived without them.

I am thankful to Harold Talbott for his unfailing wisdom and dedication in editing this book, to Robert Garrett for his mastery in making
the essence of the teachings shine through the beauty of words, and to
Lydia G. Segal for joining me in meditation for years to refine my own
experiences of these meditative exercises.

I am grateful to Daniel Goleman for his foreword, which bridges
the Eastern and Western views on the health of mind and body. I am
indebted to Ian Baldwin for his invaluable guidance in the editing and
publishing world, to Jonathan Miller for his invaluable suggestions, to
David Dvore for his computer skills, to Susanne Mrozik and Madeline
Nold for checking the Healing Buddha mantra translation, and to Vic-
tor and Ruby Lam for their apartment, so easy to work in.

My very special gratitude goes to Michael Baldwin for single-hand-
edly keeping the light of my academic projects shining and to the
members and patrons of The Buddhayana Foundation, in Marion,
Massachusetts, under whose most generous sponsorship my research
and writings have prospered for the last twenty years.

I highly appreciate Acharya Samuel Bercholz and the staff of Shambhala Publications for trusting in and caring for my book, Susan J.

Cohan for her meticulous editorial skill, and Kendra Crossen Burroughs for her insightful directions.

Whatever good comes from this book is the fruit of the ambrosia-like teachings of Buddhism. I plant them as the seeds of fruits that will heal the disappointments of all our mother beings. Whatever errors have crept into this effort are reflections of my own ignorant mind, and I pray for forgiveness from the Buddhas, the learned masters, and all my compassionate readers.

BOUNDLESS HEALING

INTRODUCTION

SINCE *The Healing Power of Mind* (Shambhala Publications, 1996) was published, I have traveled to many places in North America and Europe. During those trips, I explained the healing principles in the book and led guided meditations on healing. I also received many letters of appreciation and comments from readers of diverse backgrounds.

It is an interesting experience to be out in the world after publishing a book, especially for someone from my background. Until the age of eighteen, my home was Dodrupchen Monastery, in a secluded valley of eastern Tibet, surrounded by mighty mountains, where the routine of study and prayer was regulated by the passage of the sun and moon in the sky. The Tibet I remember when I was growing up was a timeless place, deeply religious, removed from the distractions of the modern world.

In some ways, the life I have lived for several decades in the United States is not so very far removed from that monastic existence. At home in my simple but welcoming apartment in a big city, I am surrounded by my collection of scriptures and Buddhist images, which shine forth as living artifacts of timeless truths. Much of my work has been as a lifelong student and interpreter of Buddhism, translating ancient texts so that the spark of their wisdom might take hold and catch fire in English and other languages of the Western world. I spend a lot of time alone, studying the scriptures and meditating, although I am blessed with many friends in my adopted country. Over the years, all kinds of people have come to me for advice about the struggles of their lives. This is why I wrote the first book on the mind's healing power five years ago—to talk about how we can help ourselves in our daily lives.

After that book was published, suddenly I was out of my comfortable, cell-like apartment and meeting with large groups of people from different parts of the West. All these encounters in the past few years have confirmed a belief of mine: we need encouragement in how to live. Maybe we have a dawning interest in meditation or have read a book or attended a workshop, or perhaps we have been traveling along a spiritual path for a number of years. No matter, it seems that as humans, we can always use more help. We need a teacher to point to truths that can guide us. We need to take good care of ourselves and learn how to be more encouraging and positive in our attitudes.

Most of the people in my workshops were amazingly open to the meditations, giving them their whole attention and energy. Even for those who were new to meditation or dealing with big problems, the meditations were effective and enjoyable, thanks to their dedication.

Some who were new to any kind of meditation worried about how they would be able to sit for two or three hours and then were amazed to find that the session had ended. Some experienced a feeling of spaciousness and clarity, a crack in their usual closed and tight confinement. For a while, some felt love and openness in which resentment, anxiety, dislike, or hatred could no longer be harbored. Some felt peace and strength in which attachment, craving, or jealousy had no place. Others felt that no problem was that big a deal. Even sickness seemed less significant—a passing phase in boundless space, like a patch of clouds in the sky.

In almost every workshop, there were people who politely excused themselves, having found that the attempt to meditate aroused strong resistance. Others seemed to struggle but stayed with it and did fine. Still others appeared at first to have a good experience, but because they didn't acknowledge and appreciate the positive feelings, much of the benefit slipped away.

For many, nothing seemed to work, for they were not ready to open up. Nothing could penetrate their problems, fortified as they were by rigid mental and emotional walls. It was rather shocking that some so-called experienced meditators got little benefit from the healing meditations, because they held tight to their judgments about the

2

particular approach to meditation. They appeared rooted in an attitude of pride and insecurity.

One of my most gratifying discoveries that emerged from the reaction to the first book was that anyone with an open heart appeared to benefit, no matter whether he or she was Catholic, Protestant, Jewish, or an avowed unbeliever belonging to no organized religion. A couple of people with experience in a twelve-step program for recovering from addiction were happy the book could be a source of guidance without requiring a belief in God or an adherence to organized religion. Further, Buddhism advises us to be mindful of the present moment, to let go of unneeded worries about past and future. This finds an echo in the twelve-step principle of living one day at a time.

Like its predecessor, the book you now hold in your hand is intended to benefit anyone, regardless of background. You need not practice a religion designated by the name of Buddhism to find peace and happiness, or even enlightenment. Wisdom and compassion are present in all and can shine from the heart of any being, even from the hearts of animals, as many *jataka* folk legends illustrate. The most important thing is the birth and growth of spirituality in your mind, not the ceremonial designations.

According to Buddhist scriptures, this is the reason why many self-enlightened sages (*Pratyeka-buddhas*) are able to attain the highest truth in a land and an age where there is no Buddha or Buddhism. They become enlightened by themselves because of their commitment to spirituality and their realization of the same wisdom that Buddhism offers.

Here again in this book, we are concerned not so much with the ultimate goal of enlightenment but rather with becoming happier and more peaceful in everyday life. And while some meditations using Buddhist imagery are presented later in the book, the emphasis is on a universal approach that anyone can use.

My own heritage is Nyingma Buddhism, the oldest Tibetan sect, dating back to the ninth century, when the great sage Padmasambhava brought the revelations of the Buddha from India to Tibet. Although I am initiated into the esoteric Tantric practices, I have the deepest respect for the common teachings, or Sutras. In fact, I practice many of them myself. These teachings contain everyday wisdom that is like a deep and refreshing well. If practiced with dedication, they can grant peace and contentment and even lead to higher realization. It is these

3

sources from which I have drawn, spiced with just a bit of my own knowledge of esoteric practice that I have adapted for Western readers.

People are sometimes surprised when I tell them there are thousands of meditations and practices from which to choose, depending on the person and circumstance. You could bring healing to your being just by listening to the wind or looking deep into the blue sky or watching the stars in the vast heavens above. In Tibet, the sense of spirituality was so strong that the very rivers, trees, and bushes seemed alive with sacred blessings. There's a famous Tibetan tale of a simple elderly woman who kept an old dog's tooth upon which she meditated, successfully using it as a means to realize enlightenment.[1] Of course, it wasn't the object itself but her mind's strong belief. For it is mind, above all, that is the source of healing power and wisdom.

Against this backdrop of a myriad of possible meditations, I found in my workshops one approach that seemed especially fruitful: the object of the meditation is the body itself. Now, everyone who comes to a workshop has a body, so you see right away that the attendees have what is needed to do some meditation! Furthermore, so many people are concerned about their bodies. Either they are healthy and want to remain so, or they are worried about aging, or their bodies may be sick or broken, and at the very least, they need relief from the mental anguish that sickness can cause. In Chapter 14 of *The Healing Power of Mind*, I gave a very brief description of a meditation upon the body. This present book has grown from that small seed. We are going to reflect very deeply upon our bodies in this book. The purpose is to awaken the healing energies of the body and, in so doing, awaken the mind.

While it is not always possible to cure the afflictions of the body, at least we can ease our suffering or learn to tolerate it better. In fact, a sickness can often be overcome through the healing power of mind. In the West, when people hear the expression *healing meditation*, they often put the label "New Age" on it. This is a rather strange way to look at it, and maybe a little funny from my point of view, for the principles and practices I will be describing are not so new at all but have been tested time and again over many years.

In my first book on this subject, I referred to a number of recent studies Western science has done on the benefits of meditation, and I also gave some examples of healings. It's always inspiring to hear about individual cases, so later on I'll talk about the specific meditation I used

4

to heal a difficult back problem I had. I should also mention the example of my friend Harry Winter, who, by meditating, overcame a cancer that was diagnosed as terminal. Readers seemed so interested in his story in the first book that I decided to describe again the special visualization he used (see page 43). More recently, Harry has been using another visualization (described on page 44) to overcome the breathlessness associated with emphysema.*

The question I am often asked is, What scientific proof or statistics do you have to show that these meditations can really heal problems? My answer is simple. I am attempting to present the profound, centuries-old, Tibetan Buddhist wisdom on healing in a comprehensible package that suits modern readers who are educated and open-minded but overly occupied. Each step of meditation is based on a universal, natural, and commonsense approach. If it is common sense, there is no need for complicated validation or any statistics. For example, *tsampa*, the roasted flour of barley, is the main staple of Tibetans. For Tibetans, the edibility or nutritional value of tsampa has never needed proof. I believe the issue is not the lack of effectiveness of the meditations but our lack of openness and dedication.

For hundreds of years, Buddhists, as well as members of many of the world's other spiritual traditions, have witnessed healing through the power of meditations, prayers, and aspirations. Not only ordinary problems but even life-threatening diseases thought to be incurable have been healed through the power of meditation. Also, we have often witnessed spiritual people calmly accepting sickness, prison, homelessness, or even death with smiling faces because of the peace and joy in the deepest core of their being. That is what we call the healing power of the mind.

In recent decades, Western physicians and scientists have begun to discover the great healing powers of age-old meditations and prayers. Many scientists are puzzled by the depth of knowledge attained by the ancient masters, who employed no scientific instruments. Nevertheless, there will always be many who will doubt, even though the proof is dancing at the tips of their noses.

We live in a golden age of science and medicine, even as we redis-

---

*Shortly after the manuscript for this book was completed, I received word of Harry's death due to complications of his emphysema, more than eleven years after his "terminal" cancer was first diagnosed.

cover the ancient knowledge from the golden age of the mind's wisdom. Instead of pitting these worlds against each other, we could choose to enjoy the benefits of both.

When I look out upon the earnest faces of those who come to my workshops, I sometimes wonder what they must be thinking. Perhaps they know that I was designated, when very young, as the reincarnation of a sage from another age. At age five, I was ushered into a life of prayer and study at the monastery. For some, I must seem quite exotic, but if they come expecting miracles, I hope they stay to learn a thing or two about the deep wisdom that is a birthright of us all. Some people at these gatherings may have trouble understanding my accent and my somewhat broken English. One reason for a Tibetan priest to write a book (yes, on my laptop computer!) is to make my message clearer and to cut through the cultural differences.

To be honest with you, I do not consider myself an "adept" or accomplished master. I am just a person who, like you, must navigate the sometimes rough seas of life. It is this shared humanity that I wish to emphasize. As for many of you, my life has not always been easy or smooth. I have experienced confusion and conflict, emotional upsets, and physical hardship. This was especially true when I was a refugee fleeing the political turmoil of Tibet, but there have been plenty of problems since then, too. Through all the difficult times, the guiding lights of ancient teachings have consistently helped me enjoy the wondrous gift of existence with all its challenges.

What I have to offer is not really my own but rather a treasure that everyone can share. Early in life, I was blessed and fortunate enough to be handed a legacy of unsurpassed knowledge by teachers and sages. I have many memories of the greatest of human beings, of powerful images, words, and feelings ripe with peace, love, and wisdom. These memories remain vivid and undying in my mind today. As a Tibetan proverb says, "If a piece of ordinary wood is kept in the midst of sandal trees for a long time, it will also smell like sandalwood." This is why, even if I am ordinary, I could be a vessel to bring you the great wisdom of healing.

In this book, I talk a lot about the body and the mind. But really, it is the mind that matters more. After all, sickness and death are part of the natural cycle of a life that involves the gross body and emotional mind. There is no way of avoiding illnesses forever. You have to face them when your turn comes. At such a time, the most reliable source of support is a more peaceful mind. This will help you accept and tolerate life in all its manifestations, just as you accept the cycle of light in the day and darkness at night. The third Dodrupchen, a sage who lived at the turn of this century, offers this gem of wisdom: "The meaning of becoming invincible to obstructions—such as adversaries, sickness, and evil forces—is not necessarily reversing them or preventing them from arising but not allowing them to become obstructions to our journey on the path [of healing]."[2]

Those of you who have read *The Healing Power of Mind* may be familiar with many of the principles also contained in this present book. Just as my wise teachers often repeated their advice, so, too, have I purposely done the same. This is partly for anyone who has not read that first book, but it is also because most people need repetition. They need to hear the truth again and again from others and to encourage themselves with constant reminders. I might add that the first book goes into greater detail on some healing principles and also presents many different meditations that may be applicable to your situation.

Finally, never take any healing meditation as the only solution for your problems. Problems are multiple and manifested in a variety of symptoms. Each problem is the product of numerous causes. You need a variety of approaches to your problems, including a balance of exercise and rest, wholesome nutrition, proper medicine, a clean environment, and a healthy lifestyle.

Also, different people have different healing needs. What is right for one person may not be for another. After a few days (or about twenty-one hours) of training, if you don't feel that these particular meditations are comforting, they might not be right for you, so you should seek a different meditative approach.

From the ocean of healing wisdom taught in Buddhism, I've arranged a few sips of healing nectar that my mind has tasted as a simple offering to you.

Part One

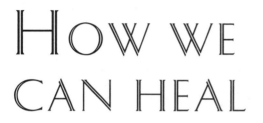

How we can heal

HEALING THE MIND AND BODY

To FIND TRUE WELL-BEING, the best place to look is close to home. We could travel around the globe a hundred times, turning over every stone on earth in the quest for happiness. Yet this would not necessarily give us what we seek. Money does not necessarily grant well-being either, nor does a youthful or healthy body. Health and money can help us, of course. But the real source of peace and joy is our minds.

The mind wants to be peaceful; this is really its natural state. But there are so many distractions and cravings that can obscure our peaceful nature. A characteristic of our time is the speed of our daily lives, especially in the West. Everything is a rush. Meditation can slow us down so that we touch our true nature. Any meditation can help us. The object of our contemplation could be a flower, a religious image, or a positive feeling. Or it could be our own bodies.

One especially rich way to develop a peaceful mind is to meditate upon the body. By doing this, we promote the welfare of our whole being.

Through meditation, we can learn how to encourage our minds to create a feeling of peace in the body. This can be as simple as relaxing and saying to ourselves, "Let my body be calm and peaceful now," and really feeling that this is happening. It is the beginning of meditation—and of wisdom, too.

This approach is a kind of homecoming. We are reintroducing ourselves to our bodies and establishing a positive connection between mind and body. Quite often, we have a rather strained and distant relationship to our own bodies. We think of the body as unattractive or ugly, or maybe our health is poor. Or else we like the body, cherish it, and foster cravings around it. But even if we cherish the body, we worry that it could be better than it is or that it will get sick or grow old. So we are conflicted and ambivalent. The body is an object of anxiety.

The meditations in this book will help us approach the body with a realistic attitude, accepting it as it is. Then we will practice how to see the body as very peaceful, a body filled with light and warmth. So many mental and physical afflictions are associated with the body, and meditation can help to heal them.

Mind and body are intimately connected, and the relationship of mind to body in meditation is very interesting. When we see the body as peaceful and beautiful, who or what is creating these feelings? The mind is. By creating peaceful feelings in the body, the mind is absorbed in those feelings. So although the body is the object to be healed, it also becomes the means of healing the mind—which is the ultimate goal of meditation.

When our minds are peaceful in meditation, there is no other mind. Even if the peaceful feeling goes away, we are developing the habit of a peaceful mind. Our minds are becoming accustomed to their true nature. Really, it all comes back to the mind. This is where our true happiness is. The Buddha said:

> *Mind is the main factor and forerunner of all actions.*
> *Whoever acts or speaks*
> *With a pure thought*
> *Will enjoy happiness as the result.*[1]

Like a physician treating a patient, Buddhism deals with mental, emotional, and physical afflictions by diagnosing the cause and treating it.

In this world of ceaseless change, the mind tends to develop a grasping quality and gets attached to all kinds of illusory wants and desires. This is at the root of our suffering. We heal ourselves to the extent that we can release that grasping.

As it was first practiced in the ninth century, Tibetan medicine viewed the body as composed of four elements—namely, earth, water, fire, and air—and as having hot and cold temperatures. Western medicine has given us a wonderfully detailed and up-to-date knowledge of the body and how it works, and we can take advantage of this. Yet even today, the ancient Tibetan picture of the body is very useful, both as an aid to meditation and as a way to understand the various qualities of the mind.

According to this view, when the four elements are in balance, we are in our natural healthy state, but when there is disharmony, emotional or physical disease can take root and flourish. The third Dodrupchen writes:

> The ancient masters said that if you do not foster dislike and unhappy thoughts, your mind will not be in turmoil. If your mind is not in turmoil, the air [or energy of your body] will not be disturbed. If the air is not disturbed, other physical elements of your body will not experience disharmony. Harmonious elements [in turn] will help the mind stay free from turmoil. Then the wheel of joy will keep revolving.[2]

The mind is the source of true well-being. So before we get to the guided meditations upon the body later on, we would do well to consider the qualities of the mind and how we can improve our lives.

THE PEACEFUL MIND

When I was ten or eleven years old, my personal tutor, some friends, and I made a rare excursion from the monastery. I looked forward to visiting the great adept Kunzang Nyima Rinpoche in a valley two days away. Though I enjoyed my life in the monastery, it was so exciting to ride a horse across the spacious Ser Valley. For miles and miles, we rode through this untainted land, enjoying the sight of peaceful and beautiful animals. Butterflies dotted the air over the green carpet of grassland, and birds played and sang freely, in a timeless scene of natural beauty. It was the greatest feast for the senses of a little boy to enjoy, an unforgettable adventure for someone who had lived for years within the sanctuary of a monastic compound.

Arriving in the evening, we reached a small, peaceful gorge walled by gentle green hills. In the distance, the majestic mountain of Ser Dzong seemed to preside over all of existence.

We camped in a beautiful field at a distance from Rinpoche's big black tent. Early the next morning, we crossed the meadow to meet Rinpoche. He had a beautiful and powerful face with wide, smiling eyes, a brownish complexion, and long hair tied around his head and wrapped in a silk turban. He might have been in his fifties, and he had a strong, vital body. With a blossoming, flowerlike smile, he welcomed us as if he had just found his long-lost friends. He kept his treasure of writings close at hand, about forty volumes, most of which were his mystical revelation. I remember the feeling of unconditional and unpretentious love in his heart, which wasn't only for me but for all around. Although his voice was powerful and far-reaching, he spoke in a stream of gentle and soothing words. He was someone who enjoyed the simple gifts of life with deepest contentment. I was a guarded and shy boy, but in the sunny presence of Rinpoche, I became so natural. There was no place to harbor darkness or anxiety anymore.

Rinpoche's joy and calm seemed pervasive. Immediately upon meeting him and for all the time I was there, the world appeared to be a very peaceful place. As I looked around, I vividly felt that his presence had somehow transformed my surroundings, that nothing was separate from this wonderful peacefulness. The trees, the mountains, my companions, myself—everything was united in calm and peace. It wasn't the mountains and people that changed, but my mind's way of seeing and feeling them. Because of the power of his presence, my mind was enjoying a greater degree of peace and joy, almost a state of boundlessness. That feeling enabled me to see all mental objects through those qualities. For a while, no attractions or disappointments mattered. Even today, when I remember that experience from more than four decades ago, I feel joy and completeness. The heat of that memory helps me to melt the ice of obstacles as they come up on life's journey.

The mind creates peacefulness. In this case, my mind had focused on an object outside itself—this benevolent spiritual teacher—and expanded the feeling of peace. We can benefit from such experiences, because they offer a taste of peace and show us how our mind would like to be. And we don't have to go to the Ser Valley to experience such peace. We can feel happier and more peaceful in our everyday lives and encourage this feeling of peace through meditation.

True healing and well-being come down to enjoying an awareness of peace, the ultimate peace of existence. The mind is not passive in the sense of being half-asleep. Instead, the mind is open to the thought and feeling of total peace. An unrestricted and uncontaminated awareness of peace is the ultimate joy and strength. When we are truly aware of peace, our nature blossoms with full vigor.

Some people are so fully open to the true nature of existence that they are peaceful no matter what the circumstances. For the enlightened mind, peace does not depend on any object or concept. Awareness of the absolute nature of things, the universal truth, is not limited or conditioned by concepts, feelings, or labels such as good and bad. A mind that is free can transcend dualistic categories such as peace versus conflict and joy versus suffering. The enlightened mind does not discriminate between a subjective or an objective reality or between liking and disliking. Time is timeless, and everything in existence is perfect as it is.

Before this begins to sound too theoretical, I should say that there are many people who are enlightened, to one degree or another. Some Tibetan lamas I know were imprisoned for many years, and they almost enjoyed the experience. I try to avoid talking about the political upheaval in Tibet, because it is too easy for blame to arise. This can lead to a cycle of resentment, which could embitter the mind and is neither helpful nor productive. Suffice it to say that prison is not necessarily a pleasant holiday. Yet I have a friend who got out of prison only after twenty-two years and had felt quite at home there because of a very peaceful mind. When I asked him how it was, he said, "It was nice there. I was treated very nice." When you ask one of these lamas to explain, he will say, "Alive or dead, it doesn't matter. I'm in Buddha pure land."

We can be inspired by tales of enlightenment, where peace is everywhere and even turmoil is OK. But for most of us, the goal should be to work with our ordinary minds and just try to be a little more peaceful and relaxed in our approach to life. If we can become a little more peaceful, it will help us handle everyday problems better, even if big problems are still difficult.

Even so, it can be helpful to remember that the enlightened mind and the ordinary mind are two sides of the same coin. The mind is like the sea, which can be rough on the surface, with mountainous waves stirred up by ferocious wind, but calm and peaceful at the bottom. Sometimes we can catch sight of this peaceful mind even in times of trouble. These glimpses of peace show us that we may have more inner resources to draw upon than we had realized. With skill and patience, we can learn how to be in touch with our peaceful selves.

THE MIND AS A SOURCE OF NEGATIVITY

If we lack peace of mind, then what good does it do us to have youth, beauty, health, wealth, education, and worldly power?

We can find many reasons to be miserable. Somehow, even if we experience some happiness or excitement, we feel haunted by a void in our lives. We all know of people who appear to have everything but fall victim to darkness and pain and even end their lives by committing suicide. Shantideva, one of the great masters of Buddhism, writes about the snares of the mind that can entrap us:

> *[The Buddha], who tells the truth, says*
> *That all fears*
> *And all the immeasurable miseries*
> *Are facilitated by the mind.*[3]

In India about twenty-five years ago, a Tibetan acquaintance of mine struggled to survive, as a lot of refugees do. After a few years, he made some money, enough so that he could live comfortably. But he never felt content with anything. From the time he woke to when he fell asleep, his mind was occupied with money. He constantly talked about money, lamenting that he did not make enough, worrying that he would lose what he had. He had no life. He was a slave of almighty money. He worried about getting sick, not for the sake of his health and well-being but because he would lose the opportunity to make a little more money. It sometimes seemed as if he were a grotesque apparition, for even his facial expression and body looked crimped, so tightly did he cling to the idea of money.

Unfortunately, he is not the only person who functions as a mere shadow cast by material goods. Many of us are more or less sucked into the same kind of existence. We take no time to cultivate true happiness and may not even be sure what that is. Many writers are occupied with mere word games and theories. Many politicians promote their ideas only to gain power. Many rich people are trapped by the drive to amass more wealth or the fear of losing what they have. Many intellectuals are blinded by arrogance or intolerance. Many spiritual teachers run a business show or go on an ego trip to gain power over others. Many poor people, in their hard struggle for survival, are unable to take any pleasure from life. The wonderful skills and achievements of the modern age often end up as fuel for greed, obsession, bondage, pressure, worry, and pain.

All these miseries could be healed by our minds, but without practice in cultivating the peaceful mind, we are too vulnerable and weak. The fault lies not with the wonderful material objects but with our own attitudes. Many of us are spellbound by our wild emotions and cravings, slave masters created by our minds. Caught up in these attachments, many of us even find it painful to be alone or experience silence.

According to Buddhism and many of the world's other wisdom traditions, the root of all our problems is the grasping of the mind. The Buddhist term for this is grasping at "self." This can be somewhat tricky for Westerners to comprehend. For one thing, the common understanding of "self" is an "I" or an "ego." In the Buddhist view, "self" includes "me" and "mine" but is also very much broader and encompasses all phenomena arising in our consciousness. However, according to the highest understanding of Buddhism, there is no "self" that truly exists as a solid, fixed, unchanging entity.

We normally think that a person is a subject who perceives and is separate from objects, and we tend to treat objects as if they were solid and dependable in some kind of absolute way. Yet mental objects—wealth, power, a house, a television show, an idea, a feeling, whatever phenomenon you can think of—are really not so absolute but instead are relative, arising and passing away, and seen only in relation to other phenomena.

But how can this be, you may ask? Surely as "I" read a "book," they both exist, since there seems to be an "I" who holds the book in my hand. The answer is that all things exist in relation to one another, and existence is marked by change. Perhaps the best way to clarify this a bit would be to use the example of the body. The body is changing all the time. In babies, we can see this more vividly because they grow so quickly. But we all know that every body changes, even from day to day—for example, according to what we eat or how much we weigh. Even our moods can affect the body and be reflected in how we look, perhaps crestfallen or haggard or else bright and vital. Above all, we know that the body ages and eventually passes away. The body is a vivid illustration of the transitory nature of existence. If we think of the body as solid, fixed, and unchanging, and cling to this notion, that is grasping at the body as "self."

To the extent that grasping at self becomes tighter, all the mental and emotional afflictions—such as craving, stress, anxiety, confusion, greed, and aggression—will be intensified, and physical and social problems will be magnified. Shantideva writes:

> All the violence, fear, and suffering
> That exist in the world
> Come from grasping at "self."
> What use is this great evil monster to you?
> If you do not let go of the "self,"
> There will never be an end to your suffering.
> Just as, if you do not let go of a flame with your hand,
> You can't stop it from burning your hand.[4]

The Buddha himself said:

> When you see with your wisdom
> That all the compounded phenomena are without a "self,"
> Then no suffering will ever afflict your mind.
> This is the right approach, the approach that cuts off all the pains of
> craving.[5]

According to Buddhism, grasping at self can be the source of physical disease as well as mental anguish. Many Western scholars agree that negative emotions, anger, and anxiety can cause many diseases. Daniel Goleman writes:

> Both anger and anxiety, when chronic, can make people more susceptible to a range of disease.[6]

How We Can Heal

People who are chronically distressed—whether anxious and worried, depressed and pessimistic, or angry and hostile—have double the average risk of getting a major disease in the ensuing years. Smoking increases the risk of serious disease by 60 percent; chronic emotional distress by 100 percent. This makes distressing emotion almost double the health risk compared with smoking.[7]

Loosening the grip on "self" is our best remedy for all problems, and to the extent that we can do this, that much happier we will be. This is healing in its truest sense. A common Buddhist scripture, or sutra, puts it this way:

What is healing from sickness?
It is the freedom from grasping at "I" and "my" [egoism and
* possessiveness].*[8]

In Buddhist scripture and commentary, *sickness* often refers to the ills of both mind and body. Vimalakirti said, "As long as there is ignorance and craving for the existents, there will be sickness in me."[9]

So much of our troubles are created by not realizing who we are and what our true place is in the ever-changing universe. The physicist Albert Einstein, pioneer of the theory of relativity, knew something about the place of the human being in the universe. While the *self* in the following quote probably was intended to mean "ego," Einstein clearly was aware of the merit in loosening the grip upon narrow-mindedness and cherished concepts when he wrote, "The true value of a human being is determined primarily by the measure and the sense in which he has attained liberation from the self."[10]

If common sense and religious tradition tell us to loosen our grasping attitudes, how can we do this? One way is meditation. In the guided meditations that come later, a primary technique is to visualize the body as filled with light, which shines outward to the universe. It can be very positive to imagine the body as boundless. This can help ease the grasping of the mind.

However, sometimes we are so mired in our suffering that it's hard to see a way out. We need to find a focus point, any positive feeling, image, or idea that can light the path before us and give us a glimpse of peace.

19

THE PATH TO PEACEFUL FEELINGS

The poet William Wordsworth said, "The world is too much with us."[11] Some of us are so busy and absorbed in worldly activity that we lose perspective on our feelings and state of mind. We cannot even bear peace or silence. We find it painful and scary not to have something active going on, such as talking, playing, digging, building, writing, counting, or worrying!

Some people aren't even aware of how unhappy they are because of their enslavement to excitement, cravings, and worries. Grasping at "self" can be like scratching at psoriasis: it almost seems enjoyable, but it only inflames the irritation. Although we have the capacity to be peaceful, our true nature has become so obscured that peace of mind is now an unknown commodity.

There's a famous story about the mother of one of the Buddha's main disciples. After she took rebirth in hell, her son, through the power of his spiritual feats, went to that realm of suffering to rescue her. He patiently gave her the teachings that could change the negative conditions of her mind. She was able to free herself from the infernal realm but was so attached to her place in hell that she pleaded with the other inhabitants, "Please don't let anybody take my place." It was not because she enjoyed the hell realm but because it was the only place she remembered or was familiar with, so she clung to what she feared losing.

It can seem daring to open the door to healing. And yet cultivating peace of mind is actually not so strange or alien. It can help if we rekindle a memory of some quiet time when no outside pressures or worries were bombarding us. Such memories give us a clue about the mind in its true, peaceful nature and can become the focus of meditation.

If we can recall a peak experience when we felt whole and complete, it's possible to bring the feelings of this recollection forward to the present. The key is to remember the image, in all its details, then expand the wonderful feeling in our minds. This memory could be something triggered by a religious experience or a meeting with a joyful person, as in the story I told about my visit with the Rinpoche when I was young. Tibetans often employ memories of their spiritual master as focal points for spiritual training, for the culture breeds a deep respect for the truly wise teacher.

20

There are so many possible candidates for such a contemplation. It could be a visit to a beautiful garden or being in mountains that are blanketed in snow or experiencing the silence of vast open fields.

One memory that has inspired me over the years took place during the difficult escape from the political upheavals in Tibet in the 1950s. My companions and I were passing through Lhasa, the capital, when we came upon some farmers tailing after their horses and donkeys on the way to market. They were singing some folk songs in their simple, natural voices. The singing seemed to rise up from the primordial earth. It had a sky-bursting quality of sincerity. I don't think any great professional singer could have surpassed the naturalness of those rough-hewn melodies sounding forth in that moment.

Perhaps my heart was more open to this beauty because I had just made a brief pilgrimage to the ancient, ageless monuments of a holy city. Whatever the reason, this felt different from other music that I enjoy greatly. It touched a deep level of my mind and awakened a state of heightened awareness in which any trace of fear or sadness melted in the air that rang with sweet voices. It is interesting, too, that this happened at a time of great change on a dangerous journey. So even during turmoil (or maybe because of it!), it's possible to taste serenity.

Happy childhood memories are another doorway to tranquillity of mind. Some of the silly and simple experiences back then gave us more joy than any of today's entertainments. I can remember at a very young age roasting sweet potatoes with some other boys in a small cave. It's an utterly simple memory but one that can fill me with a sense of warmth and freedom when I contemplate it. In childhood, the mind tends to be fresh and clear, able to feel things nakedly and intimately, before being numbed and insulated by all the excitements and burdens that come later. A day seemed to last forever then; we often felt a greater sense of space in ourselves.

If you relax and think back to those days, you might be able to remember something inspiring. This can be like discovering a beautiful piece of a picture puzzle: just coax the memory gently, and then all the details of the experience may come back.

Focus on the positive feeling and rekindle it, as if you were returning to your old, cozy home after a long and tiring journey. Allow the feeling to expand and blossom until it opens up your whole being as you are today.

It's best to choose a very positive memory or to focus only on the positive aspects of a memory. Stay with the warm feelings; rest in them until you feel complete in this contemplation. If a memory has some stain or darkness associated with it, it's possible to heal this negative aspect by bringing the light of positive feeling and energy to it.

During a pause in your daily routine, it can help to recollect or touch any warm, spacious feeling. The open quality can ease stress, as sunlight can melt away troubling nightmares.

AWARENESS OF THE PEACEFUL MIND

Peace of mind is not something we save for meditation or for the contemplation of past experiences, as if it were some special feeling separate from everyday life. We can encourage the mind to be more peaceful all the time. This is how to improve our outlook and assure our well-being. In the ups and downs of life, there is always an opportunity to cultivate an awareness of positive feeling.

When I talk about peace, people sometimes mistakenly think that this means detaching yourself from the stream of life. They view peace as if it were something strange, maybe a numbed or sleepy feeling, or being spaced-out and in a different mental zone. This couldn't be further from the truth. You can be "peaceful" when you are asleep, but that is only the absence of consciousness. The way to truly heal your life is to be awake to its simple joys and to develop an open, welcoming attitude toward all your activities and encounters with other people. You should enjoy yourself and be fully engaged in what you do.

Notice when you feel open and peaceful. Be aware of any feeling of freedom. Awareness is the key. If you are aware of peace, it has a chance to become part of your life. When you feel peaceful, enjoy it. Don't force your feelings or chase after them or stir up false excitement. There's no need to grasp. Simply be aware and let the feeling blossom and open. Allow it to expand. Stay with any positive feeling; allow your mind to relax in it. You may find your body feeling peaceful, too. If your breathing feels more relaxed, or you feel a sensation of warmth, pause to notice that as well and enjoy it.

The occasion for peace arising could be anything. It could be the sight of a toddler proudly taking a few awkward steps under the watchful eye of a parent. It could be the appearance of the evening star or the glow of the afternoon sun on the side of a city building or the soothing sound of rain in the morning as you're lying in bed. Maybe an openhearted person has said hello with a cheerful smile, or you might have freely done someone a small act of kindness. Simple activities like taking a walk or enjoying a cup of tea can grant you contentment, and even joy, if your attitude is open and receptive. Develop an attitude of appreciation.

It is possible to feel calm and joyful for no reason at all, or under challenging circumstances. The enlightened mind needs no object or sensation for peace to spontaneously arise. For the ordinary mind, however, it is better to use positive feelings as a starting place. Here's how you can do so:

- *Be aware of the positive.* At first, focus on positive situations and images and rejoice in their healing power.
- *See the positive side of the negative.* After gaining some strength in your mind, focus not only on positive objects but also on the positive qualities of negative objects. Look for the positive side of negative situations, the silver lining to the dark cloud. One excellent commonsense approach is humor, which can shift your perspective and suddenly turn a supposedly negative situation on its head!

   Many people have overly sensitive minds and therefore feel the negative more strongly, which allows anxieties to take root and grow. The remedy is to develop a less sensitive mind. You can actually decide "not to mind so much" when negative situations come up—in which case, they will be easier to handle. The third Dodrupchen writes, "If we are not sensitive, then because of our mental strength, even great pain will feel easy to bear, light and flimsy, like a piece of cotton."[12]
- *See everything as positive.* See the positive in everything, and everything as positive. Then it is possible to realize true peace beyond positive and negative. Ultimately, everything can be a source of healing, without discriminating between so-called positive and negative.

For most people, the main support of healing should be to focus on positive situations and images. However, if you immerse yourself in the positive, you can gradually but spontaneously embark on the second and third ways, first indirectly and then directly.

POSITIVE PERCEPTION

Pessimism can be so deadly. The habit of worrying about problems or seeing only the negative aspect of a situation leaves hardly any room for healing. When the mind becomes encrusted and rigid with this attitude, then everything that happens appears tainted by pain and negativity.

The mind can choose between positive and negative: it's all in the perception. A central practice in Tibetan Buddhism is positive perception. It's an approach that has proved over the centuries to yield an amazing harvest of spiritual realization as well as happiness and health in everyday life. The third Dodrupchen is a great champion of this approach. Here he explains how true healing depends not on our external circumstances but on how we perceive and use them:

> From animates or inanimates, whenever any harm comes to us, if we build a habit of identifying them with suffering, then even a small circumstance could bring great pain to us, as it is natural that whether in happiness or suffering we establish our habits, they will increase. . . . Being invincible against enemies and negative circumstances doesn't mean that we will be able to drive away all our problems or prevent them from ever arising again. But the key is not to let the problems become obstructions to our journey to the [spiritual] accomplishments. For that, we must abandon the thought of absolutely not wanting to have sufferings come to us and [instead] develop the thought of joy over whatever suffering comes to us.[13]

Problems can become stepping-stones on the path to freeing your mind. Even if you are not a great spiritual master, you can start by seeing small problems as acceptable. Try to see a difficulty as an interesting challenge. Then, if you can solve it or learn how to tolerate it, be sure to congratulate yourself on having done so. Feeling the satisfaction can bring a surge of joy, which has a positive ripple effect in the rest of your life.

A spark of peace and joy is present in every situation if you care to find and apply it. Even if you are having a hellish life, there will always be some moments of peace that you could certainly use as the source of healing.

24

On the other hand, even if you are in joyful circumstances, if you grasp at happiness, trying to hold fast to what you've got and greedily craving more, the experience will transform into the ashes of unfulfillment.

In a life of great pains, a little pain can be felt as joyful. In a painless life, even a little pain can be felt as great pain. Everything is relative, and it depends on the state of mind in which you are viewing and measuring things. In great difficulties, the hope of survival can be the focal point. Many innocent prisoners have survived torture and starvation because of the hope and belief that one day they'd be free. Hope can be a powerful focal point.

So even if your life is painful, you can find something to use as your focal point of healing, the best out of the worst situations, if you care to look for it.

Dr. Viktor E. Frankl, a psychiatrist who survived Auschwitz, counseled his patients that a kind of human dignity can transcend the most terrible real-life nightmare. His striving for meaning, tested by extreme conditions, became the guideline for his therapy practice of healing others. Frankl believed that one's attitude is a matter of choice and that affirmation is still possible under the worst circumstances, even if that means focusing on such a thought as being "worthy of suffering."

In his memoirs, published after World War II, Frankl reflects on his experiences in a concentration camp and how he was able to find the spark of hope and joy in the darkest night of tyranny:

> Somebody showed me an *Illustrated Weekly* with photographs of prisoners lying crowded on their bunks, staring dully at a visitor. "Isn't this terrible, the dreadful staring faces—everything about it?"
>
> "Why?" I asked, for I genuinely did not understand. . . . We were sick and did not have to leave camp for work; we did not have to go on parade. We could lie all day in the little corner in the hut and doze and wait. . . . But how content we were; happy in spite of everything.[14]

When I related this story in one of my workshops, a gentleman objected to Viktor Frankl's observation and adamantly insisted that any positive emotion in a concentration camp was impossible because of the unimaginable suffering. I totally understand his feelings, since concentration camps were true living hells on earth. With deep respect for this point of view, I also believe that the human mind is capable of remarkable resilience even in the most horrible situation. Perceptions and feelings are so subjective and relative. Certainly, Frankl's attitude is unusual given how dire this chapter of history was. But then, that's what makes his story so inspirational.

As one of many refugees from Tibet who fled to India, I saw a fair amount of suffering. The training in positive outlook I had been lucky enough to receive helped me through this time. For most people, it will be best to start now on a positive approach, and then if a crisis comes along in their lives, it may be easier to handle.

STEPS TOWARD BEING HAPPIER

Some people say, "I want to be happy, but I don't know how." They have little glimpses of happiness but feel unfulfilled or lonely or experience a sense of emptiness a lot of the time. The best starting point is to try to feel better about where you are right now. Cultivate an appreciation for whatever gifts life sends your way, even if they appear to be tiny.

According to Buddhism, the nature of the mind is enlightened. So your nature is good. The big problem is the negative habits of the mind, how you look at everything. These mental patterns can get quite built up and rigid, and they color and influence your perspective. Everyone has the capacity to be happy, but you have to change your mental habits and way of perceiving things.

A very good approach is to notice any peaceful feelings and encourage them, as I have already suggested. Nurture whatever peaceful and happy moments you have now and allow them to blossom.

Also, if you're unhappy and you want to be happy, that in itself could be an obstacle. It might sound strange, but a certain kind of wishful attitude could be limiting and restrictive. You compare yourself to others, which is counterproductive. Or even though you hardly know what being happy is, you keep insisting to yourself that you should have some kind of terrific happiness. It's like setting the bar too high rather than taking a gradual approach. Instead of helping you get there, it causes trouble because you can never seem to live up to some ideal.

If you can learn to be more tolerant of your unhappy condition and minimize your mind's sensitivity toward it, that in itself will become a stepping-stone toward happiness. If you don't mind as much whatever it is you perceive as painful or depressing, you will lighten your burden.

Try to reduce the degree of resentment toward the so-called un-happiness; that will be a big achievement. Change what you can to improve your situation and don't worry about what you can't change. Be more accepting of things at this very moment. Find humor or a spark of enjoyment wherever you can. That begins to move you toward greater happiness.

Don't make happiness an obsession, like some object you simply must get hold of and keep. If you can relax the obsession about happiness just a bit, then you might spontaneously become happier.

Finally, when you deal effectively with a problem, it's important to acknowledge this to yourself. In daily life or meditation, anytime you heal some suffering you have felt, you must recognize this. Such recognition can enable the powerful energy of joy to flare up. That could be a great focal point for further healing. The third Dodrupchen writes, "You must recognize that the suffering has actually transformed as the support of the path. Then you must feel a strong and stable stream of joy that is brought about by that recognition."[15]

THE INTERCONNECTEDNESS
OF MIND AND BODY

The mind is most important in determining our well-being and happiness. If our peace of mind is very deep, we can be happy even if our body is aging or sickly. Of course, we would all like to be as healthy as possible, in both mind and body. What, then, is the relationship of mind to body that people seem so curious about?

In the West, scientists and philosophers have sometimes talked about the two as if they were separate, with the intellect and thought processes distinct from the physical body. That view may be changing in recent years, as Western medical science has begun to notice a "connection" between the mind and the body's well-being.

In Buddhism, mind and body have always been viewed as intimately related. Buddhists are very interested in the mind. So if we asked a Tibetan Buddhist scholar, we could get a rather complicated explanation of mind and its various qualities, with lots of divisions and categories (six, twenty, or fifty-three).

All that is not too important for our purposes here. The main point about the mind is that there is no division between thinking in the brain, emotions in the heart, and feelings in the body. These are considered different functions of mind. Someone might cook, write, or drive a car, and these activities are being performed by the same person. In the same way, the mind feels with the heart, sees with the eyes, and hears with the ears.

The aspect of awareness is the mind. For example, if I say that it warms my heart to think about some act of kindness or a positive sentiment, both the act of "thinking" and the "warming of the heart" are the mind in various aspects of awareness. Awareness is a very important quality of the mind, and it is crucial in meditation. When we bring awareness to the body, we can call forth powerful positive energies.

There are three reasons to meditate upon the body:

1. Our own bodies are a very effective support in regaining the healing energies of the mind, since the body is so intimately connected to the mind.

2. Much of the time, the goal is to heal the ills of the body. So choosing the body as the object to be healed is practical. Meditation can be an effective remedy for these problems, depending on the skill of the meditator and the particular illness. It is also true that compared to emotional problems, physical ills can be difficult to heal through meditation, especially for a beginner. But even if our physical ills don't vanish, they can often be eased. At the very least, our minds can learn to better tolerate the woes of the body and carry them more lightly.

3. By bringing healing energy to the body, we can also improve our lives. The mind, the main actor in healing meditation, is absorbed in positive healing energies. This loosens the grasping of the mind. It becomes easier to develop a more open and relaxed attitude toward problems, including how to get along better with others.

USING THE BODY TO LEAD THE MIND

The mind is your main source of happiness, but sometimes the body can lead the way. Mind and body are so interconnected, it's important to take care of your body. If your body is healthy, it's easier for the mind to be healthy, too. You need to eat the right food, exercise, get enough rest, and try to stay healthy. But beyond those obvious steps, you can also help yourself by the attitude of the body—the way you carry yourself. Unhappiness and negativity can be held and retained in the body, in your gloomy face, your tight and tense muscles, your slouching posture. Simply by relaxing the body and shifting the posture so that it's as straight as is comfortable, you can shift your burdens so that they suddenly seem to disappear or feel lighter.

Smiling is a very simple way to feel good. It's amazing how you can lift your mood instantly just by smiling. It may sound too easy or simplistic, especially if you're someone who mistakenly believes that the wisdom of life should always be somehow obscure or unattainable, but the simple act of smiling makes uncommonly good sense. It also fits into the Buddhist practice of positive perception. By smiling, the body is giving your mind and heart a positive message. You feel more lighthearted, as if the world had suddenly become more enjoyable.

Not only does smiling lighten your outlook, but your open, cheerful face brings joy to other people. The Venerable Thich Nhat Hanh, a contemporary Buddhist teacher, advises us to smile all the time. If you are not ready to do that, you could at least smile more often. That's a good beginning.

You don't have to force a smile and actually shouldn't. Smiling takes so little effort: it's as if the muscles controlling the smile were just waiting for their chance. Notice any instant mood lift and enjoy it. It can be just a little smile; often that feels the most natural. Feel as though you have an inner smile, like sunshine within you, and that you're smiling inside without needing a reason. You may discover that your unhappy mood or mind-set is not so rigid after all.

A MEDITATIVE VIEW OF THE BODY

Your physical body is a precious treasure. It's an amazing machine: elegant, complex, and beautiful. It is also yours for a limited time. Buddhism talks about the body as a guest house for the mind and takes a quite realistic view of the body's aging and decay. Mind and body are together only for a while—all the more reason to treasure their true well-being while you can.

A common meditation long prescribed as part of monastic training in Tibet focuses on the impermanence of the body. Sometimes monks would actually meditate in a cemetery, the better for the mind to understand how ultimately unreliable and subject to decay the body is.

The focus here is simply for you to become more accepting of your body as it is. In the West, the body tends to be worshiped unrealistically. Even "perfect" supermodels seem to worry that their bodies should be better than they are, ever more perfect, and never changing. In the East, the body tends to be viewed more as something filthy and unworthy. Asians are not friends with their bodies, either. In both East and West, so much negative energy is attached to the body, and negative perception blocks the healing of body and mind. It's better to take a more balanced view.

Many people don't even want to think about their bodies. Being peaceful is so strange to them. In my workshops, they find it difficult enough just to relax and sit still. Then when I ask them to imagine the parts of their bodies, including their internal organs, it's too much to bear. Always, you should only do what you can without straining yourself. At the same time, though, a little bit of struggle isn't bad. You can learn how to accommodate yourself slowly, in a relaxed way, to what at first seems so difficult or even shocking.

By making a practice of meditating upon the body, gradually and after many sessions, you can move beyond attachment to or resentment of the body. Most people are so attached to their bodies that they identify very closely with them. It can help in meditation to see your body as boundless, like the sky. You don't necessarily get attached to the sky. The sky is there, and when you think about it, you accept and appreciate it. If you began to see the body with something like this kind of relaxed appreciation, you could genuinely approach all of life with more enjoyment.

During the meditations, we first contemplate the body and its parts. Then we visualize the body as boundless and blossoming with lovely healing energies. At this point in my workshops, people usually start enjoying the meditations a lot more!

Sometimes meditation can be enjoyable, and sometimes it can feel like a bit of a struggle. Your body may not like sitting so long, or your mind may wander. My experience is that if you are patient with your struggles in meditation, if you can relax and accept the rising up of "dislike," then obstacles tend to diminish or transform.

The difficulties can actually deepen your meditation if you stay relaxed toward them instead of resenting or fighting them. For one thing, you learn how to concentrate better rather than going off into some dreamland where everything is easy all the time. This kind of meditation eventually bears fruit. By gradually encouraging yourself, you are learning to let go of grasping. This is the way to heal yourself and enjoy a more peaceful life.

A POSITIVE APPROACH TO MEDITATION

In order to heal problems, first we must know what to do, and then we need to put that knowledge into practice. Action without knowledge is not enough. But then, once we understand what to do, mere information by itself is not sufficient, either. Shantideva writes:

> We must put [the knowledge] into practice [physically and mentally].
> What will be gained with mere words?
> By mere reading of the prescriptions,
> How can a sick person be cured?[1]

We must train ourselves in healing meditation. First, we need to decide which approach is best for us. Although there are numerous meditation methods, they could be classified into two major categories:

1. *Conceptual meditation*: An approach in which we think about mental or physical objects, again and again, in order to train our minds in a healing cycle of positive thought and feeling.

2. *Contemplative awareness*: An approach in which we may begin by focusing on a particular object, but then we unite our awareness with our meditative experience. Positive or negative qualities are not the concern so much as simply being in a state of awareness in a nonjudgmental way and merging our awareness with what we are experiencing.

The meditations upon the body in this book are mainly based on conceptual meditation and a focus on the positive. Even so, we should all devote at least some time at the end of each stage of the healing meditations to contemplative awareness, in which awareness is "merged" with whatever feelings have arisen from the exercise.

For most of us, the emphasis on positive mental objects is the most effective way of getting ourselves on the path to healing. Slowly, the more we practice, the whole wheel of our mental habits will turn more positive, and our outlook on life will improve.

A strong foundation in conceptual meditation could eventually lead us to shift the focus of our practice to a contemplative approach, so that we no longer need to rely so much on positive images. However, in this book, the focus is on the technique of positive visualization.

To that end, the mightiest weapons in our arsenal are the four powers of seeing, recognizing, feeling, and believing.

THE FOUR HEALING POWERS OF MIND

The four healing powers are positive images, words, feeling, and belief. Bringing these qualities of mind to our meditation strengthens the power to heal our mental, emotional, and physical afflictions.

POSITIVE IMAGES

When we visualize positive objects, the exercise of our imagination engages and absorbs our minds. If we can maintain the images in our minds for some duration, the healing will be more intimate and effective. The mind tends to wander about, especially if we are new to meditation. If we practice staying with the image as long as we comfortably can, eventually our concentration will improve.

Although visualization is a pillar of Tibetan meditation, many Westerners find it rather strange at first. Forming mental images is

33

universal, even if we are not used to doing it as part of meditation. With few exceptions, we all visualize constantly in daily life. Most of the time, our minds are occupied with neutral images or negative ones. If we develop the habit of seeing positive images instead, the peaceful nature of our minds begins to emerge, and we give joy a chance to flourish.

One of the practices of Tibetan Buddhism is to visualize positive images at every opportunity throughout the day, except when practical business is being conducted. We can bring meditation and its images and associated feelings into our own lives—during a short break at work, for example. This encourages the positive feelings to take hold.

Since many of us are predominantly visual, the focus is on positive images. Yet we could also use sound, smell, taste, and touch as healing methods, if more appropriate. Some people are more auditory, so they could emphasize chanting or incorporate music as part of their prayers and meditations.

Positive Words

Words can have great power, for good or ill. As thinking creatures, we constantly have inner dialogues going on in our minds. We put labels on things and name them. It is our way of recognizing and confirming the quality of something.

Meditating upon an image is made all the stronger when we recognize the image as positive and even comment to ourselves on its positive nature. For example, if we are visualizing a flower, we might think about its positive qualities: "This beautiful flower is blossoming"; or "Its color is so spectacular, the whole atmosphere is radiant with its brilliance"; or "The dew is dripping from its healthy, fresh petals"; or "It is so pure, as if made of rainbow light"; or "I wish everybody could enjoy such a feast for the eyes."

Sometimes just the conscious recognition of positive qualities is enough, without a label. But a label can help open our minds to an image, such as simply saying to ourselves, "It's beautiful," or "It's red." The point is to confirm in our minds the power of the positive. In this way, we begin to transform the negative mind-set we have built up. We can choose positive or negative perceptions. Recognizing the positive can be a strong ally in transforming our minds, both in meditation and in daily life.

In addition to positive images, we can incorporate positive sounds and scents or use gestures or touch. By recognizing the positive qualities of any of these means, we can expand their power.

POSITIVE FEELING

The mind not only thinks and recognizes; it feels. If we involve our awareness of the positive qualities of an object through emotion, the healing of mind and body is much stronger.

For example, in meditation, if we imagine a beautiful flower, we might just think, "How beautiful that flower is," but then the positive impression is a shadow of what it could be. Instead, we can open up to the flower on the level of feeling—feel the enchanting beauty, the freshness of dew dripping from it, the clarity of its colors, like immaculate light. We can feel the qualities of the flower in our hearts and bodies and celebrate the flower, instead of just thinking of it intellectually.

We can bring this same openhearted approach to appreciating the beauty around us every day of our lives. Opening ourselves to feelings in meditation can bring more zest and enjoyment to everything we do.

Generally we need to feel our emotions; it's healthy do so. But at times, we may want or need to protect ourselves from harmful emotions generated by negative situations and images. To do this, we should try to deal with the negative more at the level of thinking and intellect rather than getting overwhelmed by the emotion of the moment. We don't necessarily need to allow negative perceptions to be driven deep into our hearts at the level of feeling.

In meditation and all of life, we can bring the awareness of feeling to the positive qualities as perceived through any of our senses: hearing, smell, taste, and touch. We feel the vastness of the sky, the refreshing power of the wind, the comforting warmth of the sun, and so on.

POSITIVE BELIEF

If we do not trust in the power of our meditation to heal, its strength and energy will be weak. Belief gives the meditation a firm foundation; it engages the mind in a way that is effective and total.

This is not blind faith, but a faith and trust based on knowledge that the healing power of mind can be fully called forth with the help of images, words, and feelings. We need to believe that we actually can improve our lives in this way. Even if meditation moves us one step forward, we can fall right back if we are always harboring doubts in our minds.

Intellectual and material-minded people like ourselves can find it hard to trust and believe in anything. We need to remember that the mind is a powerful source of healing and that the purpose of healing meditation is to awaken our inner resources. We need to rely on the help of mental objects and believe in the power of the mind.

If we tend to be skeptical of everything and say, "How can I believe this will make me feel better?" it will be best to simply suspend such judgments. Even if it is only for the duration of the meditation, we should give ourselves completely to feeling and belief. Our intellects can get in the way by fighting and struggling. We may just need to take a leap into a trusting attitude.

We might think that by believing, we are only pretending to do something. If necessary, we should go ahead and pretend that we believe, but we should do so with all our heart and feeling. Remember that actors can call up emotions fully by pretending, but only if they believe in the roles they are playing.

If we can just keep seeing, thinking about, and feeling the positive qualities of the meditative object, slowly some benefits will come, though they may be simple. When we start experiencing these results, a more trusting attitude will flourish in us spontaneously.

If we like the meditation, that is the beginning of believing. We could start with just the thought of liking to visualize a particular image. As we become more familiar with the image, our enjoyment may increase. We should notice any positive feelings; that is where trust begins.

These four healing powers of mind are essential ingredients that make the healing meditations whole and perfect. Seeing images makes the healing process vivid and direct. Recognizing and designating the positive quality of images makes the meditation strong and effective. Feeling deepens and enriches the meditation and also helps us to recognize our problems, connect with them directly, and transform them. Believing is the way to perfect and confirm the healing, redoubling the strength of the meditation and its results.

By applying the four healing powers in a positive way, we can help ourselves now and also reap benefits later. According to Buddhism, the seeds of all experiences are sown in us at the level of the unconscious, or universal ground. Our mental and physical deeds, both positive and negative, accumulate in what Buddhists call *karma*.

Karma is like seeds planted in our unconscious mind, where they can hibernate, hidden in us. Eventually, karma blossoms in its conse-quences, for good or ill. Karma can take the form of physical symp-toms, emotions, or memories. Meditation with the four healing powers is a very effective remedy for a harvest of negative consequences.

The four healing powers are also applicable to daily life. We can see the positive in ourselves and around us, confirm this quality in our minds by recognizing it, rejoice in any positive or peaceful feelings, and believe in the healing power of this way of looking at the world. This approach to life can enable us to reap a great harvest of benefits.

TWO WAYS TO APPLY THE FOUR HEALING POWERS

We can actually apply the four healing powers incorrectly, so it's worth explaining the right and wrong ways.

THE WRONG WAY

A grasping attitude can spoil our meditation or dilute its benefits. Even if our meditation uses positive images, words, feeling, and belief, we can be too forceful in how we apply these qualities of the mind. We can start craving the mental image or object, straining after its positive qualities, or wanting the meditation to be better or more wonderful than it is.

Meditation can sometimes take on possessive overtones, in which we think about "how much I can get from this." We start feeling ob-sessed with results. Or we strain too hard. For example, some people look at a rose and enjoy its beauty openly and naturally. But if we grasp at its beauty in our minds, almost as if we were attacking it with our intellects or wanting to possess its beauty, then we are trying too hard.

If we continually feel tight and uncomfortable when visualizing a positive image, this is a clue that we should ease up a bit.

37

The Right Way

A goal of healing is to release stress and pressure. If we are open and relaxed, a more peaceful state of mind is possible. This doesn't mean falling asleep or being lazy or spacey. Neither does it mean being forceful or aggressive. Not too tight, not too slack: that is the right balance. We want to be awake and open so that we can give ourselves fully to the positive images and feelings.

However, if our minds are stuck in the habit of negative perceptions and feelings, even grasping at positive objects will be useful for the time being. That is healthier than continuing to grasp at negativity. If we can change our habits from grasping at the negative to grasping at the positive, it may not be perfect, but it's a step forward on the path of healing. Then, when our attachment to the negative eases somewhat, we can gradually learn to be more skillful in our meditation.

SOURCES OF HEALING

Healing meditation typically involves the visualization of light along with meditation that calls forth the health-giving energies of heat and bliss. During meditation, it may help you to visualize a particular healing image from which these healing energies are coming. This is what is known as a source of power, and you could choose any image that seems appropriate and inspirational. For example, it could be a benevolent, sunlike ball of light or a fear-dispelling flame or a cloud in the free and open sky or a sacred symbol or image from Christianity or any other religion or a powerful saint or being—anything that inspires you and taps into the power of your mind.

At the beginning of the meditations, visualize a source of power, resting long enough upon the image to feel its healing power. Then see, feel, and believe that the healing energies are streaming forth from this source to your body.

In many wisdom traditions, such images have proved extremely potent. For the secular-minded person, too, an inspiring image can bolster the mind's power.

A source of power can be very effective and meaningful. On the other hand, if you wish, you could simply call forth the healing energies from the sky above, from the air or space around you, or from your mind.

HEALING THE WHOLE BODY

The meditations in this book are focused on the body as a whole. The goal is the well-being of mind and body as well as healing or easing particular ailments in the body.

I'm sometimes asked whether it's a good idea to focus the mind on particular energy points or "channels," a technique used in certain healing traditions. Most people shouldn't attempt this, unless they are very thoroughly trained. If we properly use an energy point for concentration and the generation of energy, it could be powerful and beneficial. But given our fast way of life, with little opportunity to train ourselves, we should not try to focus on specific energy points or channels. We could overdo things or even harm ourselves.

For most of us, it's better to meditate upon the whole body in an open way. In the healing meditations, we sometimes focus on particular parts of the body, but then we always open up the meditation to the body as a whole. The emphasis is on a relaxed and open flow of energy. Such an approach is not only safe but very effective and based on time-tested Tibetan Buddhist practices.

3

BENEFITS OF
HEALING
MEDITATIONS

W HEN I WAS TRAINING at Dodrupchen Monastery, I was
helped along the spiritual path by constant reminders about the
teachings from my tutors and the scriptures. The aim was to root the
teachings quite firmly in my mind and to provide encouragement for
my journey through life. Since it can be so easy to lose our way, we all
should give ourselves positive messages and reminders.

That is the purpose of this chapter and the next one, which emphasize some points worth considering. We start in this chapter by exam-
ining the benefits that the meditations may bring and some principles
that can support us along the way.

An important benefit of any effort to help ourselves is the realization that we actually can improve our outlook and our lives. We become aware of our healing power, and that in itself strengthens it.
Sometimes the improvements may seem small. But if we focus on them
and rejoice in them, they are magnified.

Although we can overcome many problems through the healing
meditations, we cannot heal all of them. We have to get sick and die,

as that is the character and nature of life. But if we are able to generate the experience of peace through meditation and our general approach to life, then we handle problems with greater ease. This is especially true if we can cultivate an awareness of positive attitude and feelings.

Generally, we go through life with little awareness of what we are doing, let alone the peaceful and joyful nature of our lives. We mostly think about the past and dream about the future while missing what is happening right now, in this moment. If we are not aware, we are not fully living. We are like sleepwalkers or zombies. To be alive and healthy, we need to wake up. In Sanskrit, the root of the word *Buddha* is "to be awake." That is what true healing is, an awakening. As with a flower growing up from the ground and opening its petals in the sunlight, the process is generally quite gradual. Sometimes our spiritual growth seems slow and uneven. We can take a step backward or be filled with all sorts of doubts. We need to remind ourselves that the healing path is the right one to take.

GENERAL BENEFITS OF HEALING

The general purpose of healing is to improve both emotional and physical health. The healing meditations can heal, or at least ease, many different mental and physical problems:

- We may be sick because some parts or cells of our bodies are ill or dead. The healing and blessing energies can help to bring the ill cells back to health or the dead cells back to life, just as water can revive a wilted plant.
- We may be sick because the channels and arteries of our bodies have become blocked by hardened substances or impurities. The waves of healing energies can help unclog them.
- We may be sick because some parts of our bodies are broken or disconnected from the rest of the body, even though all parts of the body should function as one team. The waves of healing energies that are sent and received by every cell of the body can help all the cells to reconnect as a single team.
- We may be sick because we have lost strength in some parts of our bodies. The meditations can help us to generate and regain strength.

41

- We may be sick because we have imposed limits and restrictions on the scope and energy of our amazing bodies. These meditations can help to dismantle those confining walls and make everything boundlessly open.
- We may be sick because we have lost the memory or understanding of the true qualities and gifts of our bodies and minds. These meditations will help to awaken the memories of the true qualities of our own minds and bodies, in every cell of the body.
- Often we are sick because the elements of earth, water, fire, and air in our bodies are not functioning in harmony. These meditations will help to ease the conflicts and harmonize the elements in the body as friends again.
- Ultimately, our problems are rooted in the tight grasping of the mind, which can cause both mental and physical problems. These meditations will help to loosen the rigidity of our minds and bodies.

Peace and joy in our hearts may not heal all our problems, but they will certainly equip us to tolerate or even welcome whatever comes our way.

SPIRITUAL BENEFITS OF HEALING

The healing meditations can bring many spiritual benefits and inner realizations. If our hearts are filled with peace, then we have the greatest treasure. Grasping after money, power, youth, or beauty is simply a defense mechanism to hide our vulnerabilities. Strength lies in true peace, which is the essence of a healthy mind. If we have peace in our hearts and minds, then we can tolerate any situation. It is possible to be happy even when we are sick and our bodies are old and decaying.

The meditations are aimed at purifying the habitual cycle (karma) of negative emotions and deeds. Through meditation, we experience pure perception and bliss, the foundations of common Tibetan Buddhist as well as esoteric trainings. We learn to generate healing power and equip ourselves to serve others.

These trainings can lead to higher realization. At the very least, proper practice of the meditations will help us loosen the grasping of our minds. This is the heart of the practice, for the more we can let go of grasping, the happier we will be.

How We Can Heal

PHYSICAL BENEFITS OF
HEALING MEDITATION

Mind and body are closely related, so it should come as no surprise that meditation can help us when we are sick. Not every physical ailment can be healed, and we should realize that the body is ultimately subject to decay and death. Yet a positive and healthy mind can rouse the energies of the body to the maximum.

In Tibet, when we got sick, first we would go to a lama or say prayers for spiritual healing and then go to a doctor for medicine. We totally believed in the healing power of meditation and prayers, and when I was growing up, I witnessed the healing of many problems through their power.

The healing of mind and body is not just something exotic that only Tibetans can do. Harry Winter, an American friend of mine, used the power of meditation and positive attitude to help reverse the spread of a supposedly fatal cancer. Harry has urged me to "tell more people about this; it could help them." So as often as I can, I do just that.

In 1988, when Harry was seventy-four, his doctors diagnosed him with lung cancer and predicted that he would die in a few months. Harry had practiced meditation for years, so he already knew something about the mind's power and was prepared to deal with this crisis. He firmly believed that meditation could help him slow the disease, if not stop it, and that meditation could also reinforce the benefit of medical treatments.

To his doctors' surprise, Harry survived two surgeries, and his cancer went into remission. Five years later, when the disease returned, he decided against a third operation, which might have left him permanently bedridden. By then, Harry had become very experienced at meditating in a relaxed, open way, so during one period, he felt comfortable meditating for eight hours a day.

At eighty-five, eleven years after the terminal diagnosis, Harry is in robust health for someone his age. He has a lot of friends and a cheerful, upbeat attitude. Peace of mind has become a habit, and the warmth of his meditation has extended to his other daily activities, too.

Harry's visualization is basically the same one I describe in Chapter 8 as the alternative meditation for exercise 4, "Receive the Healing Blessings" (see page 150), in which the mind calls forth blessed nectar to wash away impurities. In his mind, Harry would see Vajrasattva, the Buddha of Purification, from whom would stream healing nectar. The nectar would enter his body from the crown of his head, purifying and healing the cancer cells and all emotional defilements. Harry always wished for these blessings to extend to all beings and the whole universe.

In recent years, Harry has also developed emphysema, which he describes as "a chronic malfunction of the lungs that makes it difficult to breathe, thus depriving the blood of necessary oxygen." After learning more about the condition—and especially about the relationship between mental attitude and the severity of symptoms—Harry created a special visualization that has given him the power to control the severe breathlessness so often associated with emphysema:

> I learned that this breathlessness, which doctors call "dyspnea," is caused not so much by the need for oxygen . . . as by anxiety, even panic, from the idea that the breathlessness might lead to suffocation. Increasing or spiraling breathlessness caused heavier breathing and greater anxiety, and so forth. Once I understood this pattern, I knew there was a remedy, at least for the anxiety and panic: visualization.
>
> I realized that breathlessness, even if heavy and apparently uncontrolled, is often a normal condition experienced by construction workers, athletes, and others. If I were one of these, I reasoned, breathlessness would not lead to anxiety, nor dyspnea. Therefore, I visualized myself as an Olympic track star, just as I had seen on TV, running as fast as possible a hundred-meter sprint. I crossed the finish line in a burst of speed. Then, gasping for breath, bent over like the sprinter, hands on knees, I breathed heavily against a background of cheering crowds in the stands, fluttering flags, loudspeaker announcements, and the grunting and gasping of other sprinters. Gradually, heavy but now seemingly normal breathing took over, without anxiety, without dyspnea.
>
> Since using this visualization, I have never [again] had the acute dyspnea that had sent me twice in an ambulance to [the] hospital.

Harry also discovered that something as simple as how we choose to define our condition—the very words we use to label the situation—can have a profound effect:

> I belong to a meditation and discussion support group for persons with life-threatening chronic illness. Members help each other

cope with their illness, and the many fears and obstructions to normal, happy living that it causes, by sharing experiences and exchanging positive, optimistic suggestions. At the very first meeting, the leader went around the group asking the participants to identify their illness. The sonorous announcement of illness after illness—lung cancer, multiple sclerosis, Parkinson's disease, muscular dystrophy—sounded like the roll call of a convocation of corpses.

At the time, I thought, "Whenever one hears the name of one's illness, it reinforces one's awareness of being sick and imprints this on the mind. The mere name itself therefore becomes an active ingredient of the illness, reminding one of being a victim each time one hears it." But there was a remedy.

One afternoon, a participant told of her many years of coping with breast cancer. Doctors had told her that it was incurable and would spread through the body, limiting her physical abilities and causing death within months. But she refused to accept this morbid verdict. Instead, she said, she decided to consider the disease a challenge. It gave her an opportunity: she could rid herself of useless goals and commitments and evolve new goals, acquire new interests and hobbies, make new friends—in other words, reshape her life consistent with the physical limitations imposed by her illness. She substituted the word *opportunity* for the word *cancer*, and there she was, ten years after the doctor had sentenced her to death, encouraging others to view illness not as a limiting affliction but as an opportunity.

For weeks afterward, whenever the word *disease* or *illness* was uttered, someone in the group was sure to echo "opportunity!" inevitably drawing a groupwide laugh and relaxation of tension. Some formed the habit of thinking "opportunity" whenever they heard or read the name of their illness, and over time, this effectively changed their outlook on life.

The life of one group member, who was suffering from multiple sclerosis, had become so restricted that she seldom ventured out of her apartment, and she feared doing anything new or making new friends. But the word *opportunity* struck a resounding chord. She had a fine singing voice, though [she was] unable to perform professionally. Now she joined an amateur group of musicians who played for free at benefits and in hospitals and nursing homes. She had replaced *illness* with *opportunity* and greatly extended her life's horizons.

The magic power of a word!

DELAYED AND UNANTICIPATED BENEFITS

If we can develop peaceful and joyful feelings, with less mental grasping, or none at all, this will result in our well-being. Even if we can't heal a particular problem, the benefits are assured one way or another, now or later. Buddhists believe that the benefits of positive action and a peaceful mind can even extend beyond this life into the next life or infinite future lives.

Like seeds that blossom unexpectedly, our positive actions can sometimes take us by surprise. When my friend Richard was admitted to a Boston hospital in December 1997 for treatment of cancer, he took with him a small picture of the Buddha of Compassion (Avalokiteshvara) and kept it at his bedside. He had a cardiac arrest during a bone marrow harvest but was saved by a highly skilled team who administered vigorous CPR.

When he was brought back to his hospital room, he still had not fully emerged from the effects of anesthesia. However, when his nurse, an Irish Catholic, asked him about the picture of the Buddha of Compassion, Richard gave her an extensive explanation of the use and significance of the image, speaking for about thirty minutes. Richard's wife, Paulette, who was at his bedside, was astonished by his conversation with the nurse.

By the time I visited him, many days later, Richard had learned about this dialogue from Paulette but could remember nothing about it himself. He told me:

> I am a Zen meditator, and I did very little devotional meditation with images and recitations. So I thought the devotional meditation I did would not make much impact. But now I know that what little I did was making a big imprint at a deeper level of my being, in my mind.
>
> What I was saying to the nurse came naturally from my heart, with little or no intellectual effort. It was something that had been ingrained in me at a deeper level. Now, when death comes, I am quite certain that my meditative results, the Buddha images and prayers, will be alive in me to transform my perceptions—pain to peace, confusion to awareness.

I told Richard:

There is a folk story from India. Once upon a time, a person lived among a particular tribal group. Though he spoke pure tribal dialect and had all their stories right, people kept detecting small aspects of his behavior that were inconsistent with that of their tribe. One day, some people decided to test him. Covering their faces and armed with swords and axes, they hid behind bushes on an isolated path and waited for him. As he rode by, they jumped out at him from the bushes, pretending to be robbers. At that moment, he exclaimed, "Oh, my God!" in the dialect of another tribal group. They then asked him to leave their tribe, as he had deceived them.

This folk story illustrates an important point: The superficial structure of our everyday culture or lives—no matter how solid it looks—is like a mirage. When it falls apart, whatever inner habits are sown at a deeper level of our mind will manifest themselves.

So if our lives collapse around us, we will be glad for whatever positive inner experiences we have generated. A big crisis like ill health can be the catalyst that brings back the peace and joy sown in our inner depths through meditation. Then it is possible for the Buddha pure lands to rise up.

4

REALIZING THE POTENTIAL TO HEAL

WHEN WE SET OUT ON A JOURNEY, we need to see where we are and make sure of our direction. Likewise, when we want to strengthen the healing of mind and body, it is good to step back and assess the state of our health and consider how to improve it.

THREE STATES OF HEALTH

The state of our health can be good or bad, of course, but there is also a third possibility—perfect health. Here's what each of these states is like:

1. *An unhealthy state:* We spend our lives embroiled in the sensations of pain, fear, sadness, confusion, and darkness. The mind and body are trapped in a constant cycle of desire and aversion. This is a state that needs to be healed.
2. *A healthy state:* We feel peace and happiness, and this experience is sustained. We should enjoy our healthy mind and body and bring

a healing approach to our lives so that problems do not overwhelm us. Even though we may be in a healthy state, as long as we are subject to the duality of conceptual existence—peace and turmoil, joy and pain, confusion and wisdom, birth and death—we are not yet in a perfect place.

3. *A state of perfect health:* We experience ultimate peace of mind that goes beyond the concepts of pain or happiness. Perfect health encompasses so-called opposites in a state of harmony, in which we accept life joyfully just as it is. In this enlightened state, it is possible to enjoy all situations in their true nature without needing to avoid or hold onto anything.

For most of us who are struggling to be healthy and happy, the points to remember here are: (1) If we are unhealthy, it is possible to heal and become healthier. (2) If we are basically healthy, we are still subject to slipping back, but the healing meditations will give us the strength, patience, and skill to regain our balance when problems come. (3) Just knowing what truly perfect health means can inspire us in our own lives.

We should remember that all things are perfect in their nature and that turmoil is like stormy waves upon a deep, calm ocean. If we know this and reflect upon it even on a conceptual level, then we will be able to accept unhealthy situations with some degree of calmness. That, in turn, will help us heal the problems we are facing and advance toward the perfect state of health.

FOUR HEALING OBJECTS

Each of us has a unique view, need, and ability. So in deciding which source of healing is best, we must choose an object that suits us. Four categories of objects can be distinguished as major sources of healing:

1. *Positive objects:* Any kind of object that has positive qualities and that we see as positive will benefit us and support healing. The object could be our own bodies, which we see as bodies of light and healing energies. It could be the open, boundless sky or anything from nature, like a river, a mountain, or the ocean. It could be any positive image or a positive taste or feeling. Beginning meditators especially need to remember that the four healing powers—seeing,

49

recognizing with words or prayers, feeling, and believing—are crucial to strengthening the benefits.

2. *Spiritual objects:* If our minds are open to them, spiritual objects possess greater significance and purer energy for healing. We could rely on any image, word, or feeling related to any divine entity, sacred place, religious person, prayer, or visualization that has spiritual significance. Buddhists believe we are all perfect in our true nature. So we could see our own bodies as a divine presence, such as the Buddha, bodies endowed with blessing energies.

   People who do not belong to an organized religion could still benefit from spiritual objects, if their minds appreciate their positive qualities. We can also "borrow" images from traditions other than our own. A Buddha image can benefit non-Buddhists, even those whose hearts are trained in warfare. In 1957, at the twenty-five-hundredth anniversary celebration of the Buddha's birth, Dr. S. Radhakrishnan, the eminent philosopher and then the vice president of India, told the following story: "A famous British general of the world wars, at the time of his death, left a Buddha statue together with a note as a bequest to another general. The note said, 'If you are in turmoil, if you are confused, or if you don't know what to do, just look at this image. It will give you some peace and some strength. It will give you some resolution.' "[1]

3. *All objects:* Accomplished meditators can use any object, positive or negative, for healing. When everything is seen as peaceful in its true nature, it is possible for every object to be a positive part of healing, whether the object be wrathful or peaceful, beautiful or ugly, spiritual or secular.

4. *The true quality of the mind itself:* For highly accomplished meditators, objects are unnecessary as a support of healing, if the mind has truly realized its peaceful nature. Such people are beyond needing positive or negative objects, because the peaceful mind is enough. Even as the physical body degenerates, as is natural for gross phenomena, its degeneration will have little or no negative effect on the mind.

For most of us, the important point to remember is that our minds are peaceful in their true nature, even if that nature is often obscured by grasping. In meditation, we can taste something of this peace that goes beyond concepts. At the end of the healing exercises, we merge our awareness in "oneness" with the meditative experience. Such an experience provides us with a way to deepen the healing of meditation. It also gives us practice in going beyond the duality of positive and negative objects, and this could also lead to higher realizations.

TWO SOURCES OF HEALING POWER: EXTERNAL OBJECTS AND OURSELVES

In seeking to heal ourselves, we can tap into two sources of healing power:

1. *The power of other people and things:* For most of us, it is very important to apply any and all available means of healing, whether it be the power of an external divinity; the power of a healer; the power of positive images; the power of medicine, proper diet, and exercise; or the power of nature.
2. *The power of ourselves:* The real source of healing is the power of our own minds. This is self-healing that comes from being what we truly are and using those qualities that are our birthright.

The true power of healing does not come from someone or something else, nor is it something that arises out of the blue. The peaceful mind is the true source of healing.

However, it is very hard for most of us to focus directly on the true qualities of our minds, so we get in the habit of relying on other people and other things. The common teachings advise us to take advantage of this habitual reliance by focusing on positive mental objects as a way to rouse the inner strengths of our minds.

Mental objects help us to heal, not because of the power of the images and words themselves but because of our minds' power to see those images and words as positive. It can be very healing to understand the truth of this. When we realize that true healing power lies in our own minds, that realization can bring us strong confidence. By knowing that we all have buddha nature, we become more confident about our inner resources. We gain the ability to be more peaceful in our minds.

When peace and joy awaken in us, we will see that their light is shining for us everywhere. If peace and joy do not dawn in us, the sunlight of peace will hardly be able to arise from any other source. As

Realizing the Potential to Heal

a Tibetan proverb puts it, "If there is no dawn from you, don't expect sunshine from your neighbors."

Praying for ourselves and others, making aspirations, and offering gifts are important ways of healing. But cultivating the awareness of mental peace and joy through the four healing powers of the mind is the most effective means of healing our problems.

THREE WAYS OF FACING A PROBLEM

Meditation teaches us about the qualities of the mind and trains us in the experience of peace. Many people think of meditation as something separate from life, but it is really not. We need to bring the positive feelings of meditation into our lives. Just as we learn about the mind in the meditative experience, we need to learn about the mind in everyday life and apply the trainings to it.

Although most people wish they never had any problems, difficulties are a part of life. Our problems teach us about ourselves, and we can use them to strengthen the positive qualities of the mind. So many of us make our problems worse by grasping at them and experiencing unnecessary anxiety about them. Just as we learn to relax in meditation, we need to carry this more relaxed and positive attitude over into life.

How we face a problem depends on the problem itself and our own abilities. Here are three ways of facing a problem:

1. *Don't sweat it.* If a particular problem is insignificant, there may be no need to pay any attention or apply any healing methods to it. We should preserve our precious time and energy for more serious issues.

2. *Avoid it.* If the problem is too fresh and overwhelming, thinking about it might only make the situation more unbearable. If that is the case, we should not think about it for the time being.

   These considerations apply not only to mental problems but to physical ones as well. With certain types of physical pain, if we dwell on the pain and become anxious, then we are adding mental pain to the physical pain and could end up feeling more negative pressure from the pain.

   We can build our strength to deal with a problem through meditation or any other positive means, such as reading, walking, or talking. When we have gained some distance and freedom from the problem, we can deal with it more calmly.

3. *Deal with it.* If the problem is worthy of attention and we are ready, then we should simply deal with it in a calm and practical way.

Learning to accept problems is a positive training for the mind. To the extent that we can, we should see problems as opportunities and challenges rather than as burdens. We could even learn to welcome problems or at least not worry about them so much, beginning with small difficulties and progressing to bigger ones. We could also see the open nature of our problems, beyond the negative labels we usually apply. If we can relax the grasping and anxiety with which we so often confront problems, it is possible for those problems to transform from enemies to friends.

THE IMPORTANCE OF A FOCAL POINT

Amid our difficulties and struggles, it can be so helpful to have a focal point. We can choose any positive mental image or experience to focus on. I encourage people to think about a peak experience and bring back the feeling from it.

One example from my own life is the spiritual experience I had on a visit to a great teacher, which I described in Chapter 1. We may find that an obviously inspiring memory springs to mind, or else we could choose from many possibilities, like a wonderful experience in the mountains or at the seashore. Even if we feel so downcast that nothing seems inspiring, we can still find some focal point to help us. Viktor Frankl, the therapist who went through the hell of Auschwitz, was able to find inspiration in the thought of being "worthy of suffering."

A focal point can be like a trusted friend to whom you can turn whether you are happy or sad. If your mood is dark or even bleak, take some time, even if it is only for a few minutes, for contemplation. Recall the image or experience, as you breathe in a relaxed way. The most important thing is the warm, open, positive feelings that come back. You can apply these feelings to the darkness of sadness, dissolving the negativity like a snowflake in water.

Depending on your needs of the moment, you can change your focal point, just as you would choose a specific medicine for a particular problem.

Realizing the Potential to Heal

THE IMPORTANCE OF RECOGNIZING
ENLIGHTENMENT AS OUR TRUE NATURE

It can be so empowering for us to understand, even on a conceptual level, that we are enlightened in our true nature. We may say, "Such a wonderful state of mind seems so far beyond me, why should I even think about it?"

The reason I like to remind people about their perfect nature is that this can encourage us. Yes, it's true that our grasping often obscures this nature. But the good news is that we already have what is needed to be peaceful and happy. By training our minds through meditation and developing the right attitudes in life, we can bring out what is already there. We can improve ourselves and be happier and healthier in our minds.

Enlightened mind is the true nature of our minds, as they are. It is the utmost peaceful, joyful, and omniscient state of the mind, free from the self-limiting conditions of dualistic discriminations and emotional afflictions. It is the ultimate nature of the mind and of every being.

The fully enlightened mind is the state of buddhahood. It is the universal nature, total openness. The enlightened mind sees things openly, without the usual duality of a subject and an object or the usual discriminations of liking happy experiences and disliking painful ones. Since everything is realized "as one," the vista of perception opens up without limits in what Buddhists call omniscience, or all-knowing wisdom. Space is boundless, time is timeless, and the restrictions of past, present, and future are recognized as mere designations imposed by the conceptual mind.

If we could realize our own enlightened minds, which is what our minds really are, at that moment our minds will become truly free, without the usual grasping or slavery to mental objects. All phenomena will arise and function harmoniously, not separately or as opposites.

It seems foreign to us, a mind that always remains at peace and enjoys such high wisdom. Even harder to believe is that we all possess enlightened minds.

Here we must remember the many fully enlightened ones, such as the Buddha, who cared for neither name nor fame nor prosperity nor anything except the truth, and after realizing the true nature of mind, taught this to us in the scriptures. Thousands of great sages of many spiritual traditions for tens of centuries have experienced more or less the same truth, and many people today are enlightened to a greater or lesser extent.

I have already explained in Chapter 1 how most of us glimpse the peaceful nature of our minds during quiet times when we feel centered and happy. We also can remember times in childhood when our minds were less crowded with their own creations and events than they are now.

When I talk about enlightenment, I also like to mention the phenomenon of "near-death experience." The stories people tell about what happened to them when they passed temporarily out of life are amazingly similar to centuries-old Tibetan Buddhist teachings on dying. Tibetans are fascinated by such stories and call people who have had these experiences *delok*, or "returners from death."

Many characteristics of near-death experience are significant in what they tell us about the nature of the mind. At the time of dying, people often feel themselves coming out of a tunnel, where they encounter an amazingly bright, peaceful, blissful light. Then they merge in oneness with the light and the feelings of bliss and peace. Although the experience is often described with words like *bliss* and *peace*, those who have gone through it say that the experience is beyond the realm of what can be designated by words.

These returners from death often recall seeing or reviewing their lives in a couple of minutes, with events from childhood to death not seen one by one but experienced simultaneously. They did not need to see objects with their eyes, hear sounds or words with their ears, or experience feelings with their bodies, for they perceived all the forms, sounds, and feelings in an awareness that was clear and open. This is similar to the quality of omniscience of the enlightened mind.

Quite normal, down-to-earth people have reported these "enlightened" experiences during their close encounters with death. So the enlightened mind is not a strange or foreign thing but the true nature of us all.

It's also interesting that these experiences happen just at the moment when a person is passing away from the body. It is good to do what we can to maintain our health and live a happy life. But then the day comes when it is time to let go of our cherished body. Just when we stop clinging, a blissful state can arise. Maybe we can learn some-

55

thing from the "letting go" that can come in dying and apply this lesson to our behavior in life. Why wait until death to stop clinging? We can stop right now or at least learn to soften and loosen our grasping attitudes. That will make us happier and give joy a chance to arise in us.

5

ENCOURAGING OUR MEDITATION

BEFORE BEGINNING THE healing meditations in Part Two, it
will be helpful to consider some logistical issues and tips on how
we might encourage ourselves in meditation.

SOME PREPARATIONS

Sit in the right position. Sit in a way that helps you feel physically at ease
and mentally alert. It is helpful to keep the spine more or less straight
and to hold the upper body erect as if you were pulling it up slightly.

If your spine is straight, your breathing will be natural, the flow of
energy will be unimpeded, and your mental functioning will be unhin-
dered. If you are sitting on a chair, the soles of your feet should rest
flat on the floor if possible. It helps you to be grounded.

It is not beneficial to lean against anything unless you need to. Do
not keep any object on your lap, as it could cause a subtle distraction.

Decide whether to keep your eyes closed or open. It is better to keep your
eyes open, because this facilitates clarity and wakefulness.

If you are not an accomplished meditator, however, then it will be easier and more appropriate to keep your eyes closed, as this will prevent you from seeing any distracting physical objects or movements.

So your eyes can be open or closed, depending on your needs. If you choose to meditate with your eyes open, try keeping them half open and looking into space about two feet beyond the tip of your nose.

Relax the muscles. If you feel tight or tense, slowly and gently tighten all the muscles in your fists and then the muscles of your whole body. Then release them with a feeling of relaxation in the muscles. Enjoy the feeling of relief from the tightness and repeat this a few times if you like.

Breathe naturally. Breathing normally and naturally is a great support for meditation. The relaxation can be deeper if you relax your stomach muscles, so that the breath comes freely from the area of the diaphragm. Also, it is relaxing to keep your mouth slightly open, even if you are breathing through your nose.

Breathing techniques vary according to the purpose of your meditation, whether it's to foster a contemplative state or to encourage the movement of energy. Mostly, you are interested in natural, relaxed breathing that promotes a calm mind.

If your breathing feels stifled or uncomfortable while you are meditating, do one of the following exercises:

- Concentrate more on two aspects of the breathing, inhaling and exhaling, with the inhalations shorter and the exhalations longer. Or count your breaths. An especially relaxing exercise is to simply focus on your exhalations. This releases tension and frees up the breathing.
- If your breathing seems constricted, bring your awareness to the feeling of the breath's being held back or blocked. Don't try to do anything about it but just be in touch with that feeling. Then exhale a deep breath and think and feel that the constriction is entirely cleared, and all blockages are totally blown away, like unclogging a faucet. Feel and believe that your breathing is now moving naturally.

In the guided meditations, you will be learning a breathing technique that sends waves of healing energy to the body. This is a marvelous way to move the breathing freely and to open your mind and body to healing.

SOME TIPS FOR MEDITATION

During meditation, if you experience uneasy sensations—pressure, stress, suffocation, worry, or pain—you could use any of the following exercises that you find appropriate:

- Take a couple of deep breaths and expel the sensation of worry or discomfort with the outgoing breath. Feel the peace.
- With the outgoing breath, send the sensation far away in the form of dark clouds that dissolve into the open, empty, clear sky.
- Think of the word and feeling of "boundlessness."
- Think and feel that your body is boundless, that even its cells are boundless. Allow your breathing to relax in the boundless feeling, as though your breath were totally free and without limits or constrictions.
- Think and feel that all the cells are breathing, in and out, directly through the pores of your body.
- Imagine your body as if it were a body of light. Light is intangible and free. Feel what that would be like.
- Be aware of any uneasy sensation in an open way, without judging it and without wanting to push it away or cling to it. Continue to breathe naturally and remain in the state of mere awareness. Open awareness is considered a high form of healing and can help anyone, during meditation as in the rest of life.
- If you feel as if you were floating, imagine that your body is filled with light that somehow has a heavy quality. Although light is insubstantial, we could think of it as heavy, the way air is weighed down by moisture or the way the earth's atmosphere exerts air pressure. Or just remain in open awareness of the floating sensation, without judgment, worry, or grasping.

DURATION OF MEDITATION

People often ask me how long and often to meditate. No one way suits everyone. Spending more time is better, but it depends on the individual's needs and potential. If you have demands on your time and energy, then the effort to meditate could just create more of a burden.

So you should meditate as much as you can but only for as long as you feel comfortable.

Generally, training in meditation begins with a phase in which you introduce your mind to the practice. After you have laid a good foundation, it is a matter of maintaining and refreshing your habit of a more peaceful mind.

In the introductory period, two approaches are possible:

1. If you are meditating in a gradual and relaxed way, it might be important to practice for at least a couple of hours every day for a couple of months.
2. If you are meditating more intensively, it might be appropriate to meditate for many hours every day for a couple of weeks. If you have never meditated before and find yourself struggling, the gradual way might be better.

When you are maintaining your practice, it is best to meditate every day or at least every other day. Otherwise, you will lose the continuity you have achieved by your previous meditations. Spending more time is always better, but practicing for thirty minutes or so every day or every other day ensures continuity and increases the healing power of meditation.

Whatever your experience, if you meditate for hours, take short breaks of five minutes or so every half hour or hour. It will help you keep alert, clear, and energetic. During breaks, don't get involved in distractions such as talking with people or watching TV. Instead, do something that eases any mental or physical fatigue caused by sitting and concentrating. You could look at the open sky, breathe some fresh air, enjoy a couple of sips of water or tea, or do some simple stretches.

During meditation, you shouldn't put any pressure on yourself, rush to finish this and that, or become mechanical. With a relaxed mind, let the meditation unfold at a natural pace, like the flow of a stream through a wide open plain.

OVERCOMING RESISTANCE

When we start to do something meaningful and important, such as meditation, excuses always come up that prevent us from giving it our whole heart and attention.

How We Can Heal

We can fritter away days and nights on mindless diversions, but when it comes time to meditate, suddenly all sorts of obligations, false expectations, or doubts arise. We might think, "I should be with my family," or "I need to concentrate on making money," or "I should be doing some social work." Or else we doubt the meditation: "I'm not equipped for this. Maybe there's a better method," and so forth. The self-deluding excuses are endless.

Obstacles like these, both in daily life and in meditation, can start as innocent imps but turn into destructive demons if we are not careful. A few years after arriving in India as a refugee, I began to learn English. Whenever I picked up my English reader, my concentration was always broken by such thoughts as, "It's more important to pray and meditate than to study English. Before I can learn English, I might be dead. At death, nothing but positive habits of mind will benefit me." But then when I prayed, messages would come into my head, such as, "Life is long, refugee life is hard, and in order to survive, I must learn English."

I indulged in all kinds of feasts of laziness to avoid what was good for me. It took a lot of time and effort to overcome my resistance and to feel comfortable learning English when I was supposed to study it and saying prayers when I was supposed to pray.

Overcoming such habitual tendencies, reprogramming my mental habits, came as the result of long and consistent discipline through two methods: (1) vigilant mindfulness and (2) applying the whip of right messages.

Mindfulness is the term Buddhists use to describe the giving of oneself to the moment. Instead of worrying about the past or planning for the future, we learn to feel at home in the present. It is the most wonderful guardian of our well-being if we live this way. So, no matter whether we are cutting the lawn or meditating, we should give ourselves completely to that. Our minds are really most at home living fully like this, but it can take practice before we learn to be in the present moment without chasing after cravings or worries.

If we feel resistance to something, one approach is simply to be aware of the resistance, without judgment or guilt. Then we can ease into the activity slowly, with an openhearted feeling that we will simply give ourselves to doing that. It's surprising how much we can learn to enjoy what we're doing if we are patient and open and if we just live in the present.

It could also help to push ourselves a little, gently but firmly. We can recognize the tricks of the wild and wandering mind and give ourselves a positive message to get back on track. When I was growing up in the monastery, my wise and dignified tutors knew all the tricks of boys who could be lazy and unruly. Often teachers could be strict, but my teachers were always loving. Sometimes the training we give our minds is like the training loving parents give to small children, who must be guided to keep them from wandering off into possible harm.

We need to learn a balanced approach to our minds, sometimes pushing gently but firmly if the mind is too lazy or wandering but never being too forceful or aggressive. When we are meditating, it can be easy to give up at the slightest unpleasant feeling or resistance. Again, we should simply be aware of those feelings and then ease back into the meditation.

FEELING GOOD ABOUT MEDITATION

Many beginning meditators have complained to me, "It isn't fair for me to meditate in a pleasant place and experience peace while so many others are struggling."

Although this is a beautiful thought, it is also outrageous. If we are honestly worried about being selfish, we are to be commended for such a wonderful attitude. If we respect and care about others more than ourselves, that is the heart of Buddhist practice. That attitude will naturally give us more strength and openness, and those who have it deserve to be saluted. But most of these guilty feelings ("I should be helping others, not meditating") are excuses to avoid making a commitment to anything worthy. Those who dwell on the need to be "selfless" as a substitute for nurturing peace of mind may be using this as an excuse to remain idle.

Such guilt feelings could be a sign of shock, a reaction to having our inner wounds poked by our new experience of meditation. The experience might be so intense and foreign that some of us feel safer shying away from it than bearing it.

We must understand that in order to help others, we need to improve our own minds and allow ourselves the chance to experience peace. If we don't have bread, how can we share a piece of bread with another hungry person? If our minds are filled with worries, hatred, and pain, how can we help others find peace and joy?

As the Christian contemplative Thomas à Kempis said, "Keep yourself at peace first, and then you will be able to bring peace to others."[1]

MAKING IT SIMPLE

Sometimes a very simple approach to meditation is needed, either because of time constraints or because utter simplicity suits your temperament and background.

One of the simplest meditations of all is to follow your breathing. Bringing your awareness to your breathing is an elemental act of contemplation. It focuses and calms you, and while it is absolutely appropriate for beginners, it can also lead to higher realization. During the activities of the day, you can reconnect with your breathing at any moment, touching calmness and peace on the inhalation and exhalation. When you are distressed, focusing on the exhalation can help calm you down.

Another simple approach is to meditate on first waking in the morning, while still in bed. When people are looking for something "easy" but effective, this is the practice I most often recommend. Your awareness is so open upon first awakening, it is a fertile moment to encourage your peaceful mind. Instead of chasing after scattered thoughts and worries, simply rest in the open feeling of waking up. Be aware of the warmth of your body or your breathing or the light coming in the window. Rest openly in whatever feeling you are having. You could also think of your body as being a body of light, like the light of a new day.

When you rise, get up mindfully, with a heart open to the new day. Then pause during your daily routine and bring back whatever peaceful or spacious feeling you may have experienced in the morning. Allow yourself a few moments to rest in the openness.

You need to know enough about your mind to choose which meditation is best suited to your needs. Your needs, as a meditator and participant in life, can change according to the moment and the demands of mood and circumstance. The wise counsel of others can help you. But ultimately you are responsible for your own well-being and must look to your inner wisdom to help guide you.

AVOIDING EXPECTATIONS

For healing, it is important to have inspiration. A hopeful and inspired feeling generates enthusiasm, trust, and openness and makes it easier for us to meditate.

However, we should not obsess about the meditation experience or have rigid expectations about what should happen. Grasping after results will only become a tourniquet that constricts our mental and physical energies.

We shouldn't impose mental limits of time, quality, or scope, such as the thought, "I should be healed within such and such a time," or "I must do an effective job of healing my problem." Such a mind-set can limit our progress.

In a natural way, we must take every breath and every day of our lives, no matter what it brings, as part of the process of healing, just as people go to work every day, rain or shine.

STAYING WITH IT

Some people who come to my workshops think that all their problems will be cured, like magic, in one session. Unfortunately, it hardly works that way. These days, we're conditioned to want a "quick fix" and instant results. If we meditate with wholehearted openness, it can make a difference even in a weekend. But we have to keep going.

Not long ago, a great Buddhist spiritual teacher gave a talk to a Western audience, advising them to meditate a little bit every day. "It may not make a difference in the short run," he said, "but in weeks, months, years, or maybe decades, then you will feel something different." People started laughing; they had wanted to hear him say that all the benefits would be achieved immediately. But it can take time, and that discourages a lot of us. If we resolve to practice this week for ten hours and we're not totally changed people as a result, we're ready to give up. We think it's not working.

For years, much of our energy has gone into worrying about problems and about what we want. This is like negative meditation. So we've been training ourselves in the wrong direction. Reversing this takes more than a few hours or days.

We need to be patient and consistent. We eat food every day. We don't question doing that. But when it comes to meditation, we somehow think, "I did it once; I don't want to do it again."

The key is to make meditation a part of our lives, like weaving a thread into the fabric of a tapestry. Bringing an attitude of enjoyment to our meditation helps tremendously. It also helps for us to bring the peaceful feelings of meditation into our daily activities. That is how we can begin tasting the fruits of our efforts.

When the healing of mind becomes a habit, our minds become like a great river. Although the river may not always appear to be moving, if we look closely enough, we will see how the water is slowly, slowly making its way to the sea.

REJOICING IN PROGRESS

It is always important to see and recognize the progress that you have made as the result of your meditation, even if it is small. Notice any positive change in how you think, feel, or act. Give yourself the opportunity to enjoy the experience of feeling good, as much and as long as you can. Celebrate and rejoice in any progress whatsoever. When you stumble, be glad of that, too, since struggle can be a fruitful part of growth if you think of it that way.

Even if you have made good progress, you will diminish it by thinking, "Oh, my meditative progress is so insignificant," or "What can a little meditative experience do in relation to the mountains of problems I'm facing?" Then the positive energy that you have generated by the meditation will dissipate, and your negative energies will have a chance to regain their foothold.

If you meditate for five minutes, don't say, "It's too bad I couldn't have meditated for half an hour." Instead, tell yourself, "I did five minutes. Wonderful!" Sometimes we are lazy, crazy, or wild; then we may need to push ourselves back on the path. But beware of always putting a negative spin on what you do. Instead, notice the positive, expand on the feeling, and keep the healing energy flowing.

When you rejoice over the meditation that you have done, then even if your meditation and its results are insignificant, the healing power generated by them will become magnified. The healing of your afflicted mind can continue day and night because of the power of rejoicing. It is like investing a little capital in an extremely hot stock in a booming market.

Part Two

HEALING MEDITATIONS ON THE MIND AND BODY

6

THE GUIDED
MEDITATIONS

INTRODUCTION

The heart of this chapter consists of twelve meditative exercises, three of which include optional versions that can help you deal with special needs or circumstances:

1. Bring Your Mind Back to Your Body.
2. Scan the Anatomical Details of Your Body.
3. See Your Body as Made of Infinite Individual Cells.
4. See Each Cell as a Cell of Light.
5. See Each Cell as Vast as the Universe.
6. Feel That Each Cell Is Filled with Healing Energies.
7. Heal Your Body with Waves of Light and Energy. (*Optional:* Perform a Special Meditation to Heal Proliferating Sick Cells.)
8. Hear the Healing Sound of AH.
9. Open to Healing with the Blossoming Lotus Movement. (*Optional:* Open to Healing with Other Movements to Relieve Physical Ailments and Promote General Health.)
10. Share the Healing Waves with Others.

11. Share the Healing Waves with the Whole Universe. (*Optional:* Protect Yourself with a Healing Aura.)
12. Rest in Oneness with the Healing Experience.

Before you begin the exercises, though, you might wish to give some thought to how you will perform the various stages of the meditations and the visualizations they involve. The next two sections offer some brief suggestions for how to find the approach that works best for you.

KNOWING YOURSELF AND YOUR NEEDS

Meditation is a way of training yourself to develop a more peaceful mind. Everyone has different capabilities and needs when it comes to this training. You don't want to push yourself or be too forceful, but you also want to avoid being slack or lazy. You need to develop a sense of what's best for you.

When you are new to this training, it takes some effort to go through the visualizations. This is similar to what happens when you first do any kind of physical training; it can seem difficult initially. But often it gets easier as you proceed, because your body becomes stronger, just as your mind becomes trained after meditating for many sessions. You're able to concentrate better and call forth peaceful feelings and healing energy more easily.

It's best to familiarize yourself with all the stages. This deepens your ability to bring healing to mind and body. Later, you can focus on the stages that are most relevant for you. For many people, the focus will be on generating healing waves, but it depends on you and what you need at a particular time. For example, if you are feeling emotionally stifled or rigid, meditating on your boundless body can help. Maybe in a particular circumstance, you would do only that meditation. You are in charge of your own welfare, so you can design your meditation to suit your needs as they arise.

All the same, if you only do what you want or what's easiest in life, you're likely to miss a big opportunity to help yourself. This is why it's good to achieve a balance. Do what you comfortably can but also be open to expanding your abilities.

If you are new to these meditations on the body, concentrate on the first stage (in which you bring your mind back to your body) by

Healing Meditations on the Body

itself. When you feel that you have gained some solid experience with the unique qualities of this stage, then you are ready to add the next exercise. Step by step, you should add the other stages, according to how you are progressing. If you feel stress and strain from what you are doing, you need to wait before adding the next exercises.

Once you are familiar with all the stages of the exercises and are enjoying them, you should meditate on them all in every session. You can tailor the exercises to your needs—simplifying, abbreviating, or eliminating some in a particular session and focusing on others.

For inexperienced meditators, the first stage is especially important. For experienced meditators, it is sometimes enough to simply take a few breaths, relax, and generate calmness. The mind that is very used to calming the body knows how to be in touch with that feeling.

Two of the stages deserve special attention: exercise 6 (in which you call forth healing energy) and exercise 7 (in which you generate healing waves). You would do well to build your practice mainly around these. The exercise on healing waves is especially powerful.

Many people find healing with movement or gesture (exercise 9) very powerful, too. The final stages, 10 through 12, are the natural culmination of the entire series of exercises and should be considered essential. These are the stages in which you share healing with others and with the universe before finally resting in "oneness" with the meditative experience.

SEEING THE DETAILS

The guided meditations in this chapter are quite detailed. Remember that the level of detail you see depends on your experience and the needs of the moment. Although more detail is better, the rule is always to do what you comfortably can without being overly forceful. It is important not to try so hard that you are mentally grasping at images and feelings with attachment or craving. Give yourself fully to meditation in a relaxed and open way.

In the various stages of meditation, it can be very helpful to progress through each part of your body one by one. This enriches and deepens your meditation. Yet if you have a firm foundation of experience, or if your time is limited, you don't necessarily need to do this. For example, visualizing that your whole body is radiant with light can be enough, without needing to see each part of your body.

71

On the other hand, you may prefer to go into even greater detail, as a way of deepening your meditation. In stage 2, you will learn how to scan the anatomical parts of the body. In stages 3 through 9, you could incorporate anatomical scanning into each exercise. For example, when you meditate upon the healing energies of heat and bliss, you could bring these energies to each anatomical detail of the body and its organs instead of merely seeing generalized parts of the body.

However, sometimes you may need a very simple meditation. Meditating on the whole body as radiant with healing light is both simple and very healing. Even during a busy day, you could pause and see your body this way or touch upon other spacious feelings generated by the healing meditations.

THE TWELVE STAGES OF MEDITATION

Each of the following exercises opens with background information about that stage of the meditation, followed by detailed instructions on how to perform the exercise in a way that could deepen your meditation. In practice, you will eventually combine all the exercises, or as many as you comfortably can, into one meditation.

1. *Bring Your Mind Back to Your Body*

You probably feel that your mind and body are basically functioning in harmony. After all, your mind is part of your body; they're interconnected. But often mind and body are not truly communicating. There's a dysfunction, similar to when members of a family relate to one another in a distant way even though they live in the same house and should be on intimate terms. Instead of body and mind functioning together in a protective and nourishing way, there's an estrangement. Instead of positive energy flowing through body and mind, the energy is negative or blocked. You need to bring your mind back to your body.

Meditation is a wonderful way to help you do that. In this first guided meditation, you will learn how to calm your body, pacify uneasy sensations or negative energies, ground the floating mind, and finally, feel peace of mind and body. When the mind and body are reunited, you will have planted the seed that prepares you for deeper meditation.

If you are upset and in turmoil, you may need to dispel uneasy sensations before you can become calm. During my workshops, I explain a meditative technique to do this. Very simply put, you visualize a dark cloud inside the body that contains the negative energy. Then you send the cloud off into the sky, where it disappears.

Often, someone expresses concern that this sounds as if, mentally, we were polluting the atmosphere by dumping our impurities outside ourselves. Having such a concern may indicate an overly sensitive mind, but in any event, the issue is easily answered. If you harbor and cling to your mental, emotional, and physical impurities, you are already polluting this planet. By sending the cloud away and dissolving it into the empty, open sky without leaving any trace, you are purifying yourself and the earth. It is better to recycle and completely dissolve the garbage than to pile it up at home.

Purpose: Calling the mind back home to the body brings you a feeling of peace and calm. When the body is calm, the mind is calm. When mind and body are at peace, you are calling yourself back to your true nature.

The calm you feel will help produce stability in your mind. It then becomes easier to meditate, to focus on whatever you like. In this case, you will be focusing on the next eleven meditative exercises on the body. The goal is a calm and healing mind, a mind that spontaneously manifests healing energies that permeate your body—and your life.

❀

This meditation is intended to call your mind back home to your body. The main focus is on "bringing calmness to your body," along with "being at one with the feeling of calm." Two other exercises are described to help you deal with any uneasy sensations or moods.

You could repeat any of these exercises as many times as you need to in a session. Once you have gained a firm sense of calmness, you may not need to meditate by going through the body part by part in every session of meditation.

Bringing Calmness to Your Body. Your mind can create a feeling of calm. So let your mind generate calmness in your body by thinking, "Let my body be calm." Think and feel that your whole body is calm. Give yourself permission to feel very calm and relaxed.

Now slowly go from one part of your body to another, deepening the feeling of calm. Start with the soles of your feet. Bring awareness of calm there. Then expand this feeling of calmness to your feet. Actually feel that your feet are calm. Go on slowly to your legs, your abdomen, your upper body, your shoulders. Feel that your arms and your hands are very calm and bring calmness to your neck. Feel that your head is calm. Bring awareness of calm to your brain, which is usually so busy with thoughts and plans. Enjoy the feeling of calmness and peace there.

Spend as much time at each part of your body as you need, bringing an awareness of calm there. If you feel any areas of tension—for example, in the muscles of your shoulders or neck—simply bring awareness to those muscles; tell them it's OK to let go and feel completely relaxed and calm.

When you feel complete in each part of your body, bring your awareness to your whole body again. Enjoy the feeling of your body's being one in deep calmness and peace.

Now think and feel that everything around you is also calm, as if an aura of calmness were filling the room. Now expand that feeling to the town, the city, or the countryside where you live. Now feel that the whole nation is filled with calmness. Expand that feeling to the whole earth and finally the entire universe. Everything is calm and peaceful. Enjoy the feeling of boundless calm and universal peace.

Dispelling Uneasy Sensations. If you are experiencing any uneasy sensations—such as boredom, suffocation, worries, pressures, or pain—then use the following meditation.

With a calm disposition, feel and acknowledge the presence of the uneasy sensation and recognize its particular quality. See where the sensation is located in your body, such as in the stomach, chest, or head.

Visualize and feel that all of the uneasy sensation has gathered in the form of a dark cloud at the place in the body where the sensation seems to be centered. Without grasping at it or pushing it away, briefly touch that dark cloud with your mind, feeling the uneasy sensation that you have recognized, making sure it is gathered up in the dark cloud.

Now take a couple of deep and forceful breaths and expel the dark cloud with your outgoing breath. Out loud, or silently in your mind, with each expelling breath, say, "Haaa! . . . Haaa!! . . . Haaa!!!"

Now visualize, feel, and believe that the dark cloud with its uneasy sensation has been totally expelled from your body, leaving no trace behind. Take a moment to enjoy the feeling of your body. Feel that it is free and calm.

Visualize the dark cloud as hanging in front of you, in space, a couple of feet away, still blazing with the energy of the uneasy sensation. Now see the cloud floating slowly away, through space, like a balloon drifting off. Keep watching the dark cloud float and feel that any uneasy sensations are floating away with it. Allow any uneasiness to drift away. The farther the cloud floats from you, that much freer are you from the energy of the uneasy sensation, as if you were walking away from the heat of fire. Recognize whatever feeling of relief you are experiencing.

Visualize the dark cloud as becoming smaller and smaller, like a bird flying away at a great distance. Now the dark cloud has floated miles away or even hundreds or thousands of miles away. You are totally losing connection with the dark cloud and feeling of uneasiness. At the farthest horizon, the cloud becomes as small as a tiny dot. Finally, it completely dissolves without a trace.

Keep looking at the place in the clear, open sky where the dark cloud has totally evaporated. Enjoy the openness and purity of the sky, with no trace of the cloud.

Allow your mind to touch the freedom of your body, which no longer harbors the uneasy sensation. Relax in that feeling. Let your body feel newly awakened calm and peacefulness, without worries or pain.

Grounding the Floating Mind. If you are feeling scattered, anxious, or jittery or experiencing any other floating sensation, you can ground your mind by bringing your awareness to the touch of your body on your seat. Forget all other mental objects and feelings. Just feel the touch of your body on the seat.

Now think and feel that you are not only sitting on a chair or a cushion but that you are firmly seated on the earth. Feel the touch of your body on the earth. The earth is firm, solid, heavy, unmovable, and unshakable. Feel these qualities of the earth's energies.

Feel not only that you are touching these earth energies but that your body is also being filled up with them. Your whole body feels firm, solid, heavy, unshakable, strong, and unmovable. Feel that you are united with these positive earth energies and that your body is now firm and calm.

For grounding, you could also visualize a heavy golden statue of the Buddha or a majestic mountain of rock. Feel the heaviness of the object, again and again. Then relax in open awareness of the heaviness.

Another grounding technique is to breathe naturally, with the air passing through your respiratory system. Then hold a little breath at the bottom of your stomach, a little below the navel, by pressing down slightly and pulling up slightly.

Note: During any of the stages of healing meditation that follow, if you feel uneasy sensations and need to restore calmness, you can use either of the preceding exercises in their entirety or in an abbreviated form.

Being at One with the Feeling of Calm. When you feel complete in the exercise of bringing your mind back to your body, notice and enjoy any feeling of calmness in your body as the result of meditation.

Then just relax in the state of open awareness of the calm feeling, without grasping at it or analyzing it. Let yourself merge with the feeling of calm and remain in oneness with it, in total silence, like water merging with water.

2.   *Scan the Anatomical Details of Your Body*

In this exercise, you will look within the body in as much detail as you can. By doing this, you are connecting with the body. With your mind's eye, you'll visualize, or "scan," your head, upper body, arms and hands, abdomen, and legs and feet.

Some people have trouble with this scanning exercise; they don't like to think about the inside of their bodies. You should try to see as clearly as you can the various parts and organs of the body, to the extent that you know what they look like. (The accompanying illustration on page 78 will help to refresh your memory, particularly about the internal organs.) Remember that it can be beneficial to push yourself a little bit. You may be surprised that you can push your limits, in a relaxed way, in how much you see of the body. If you come to terms with your body below the skin, it helps you develop a more accepting attitude toward your body. That attitude carries over to the rest of your life, making you happier and more accepting of yourself.

But push gently, not forcefully. Don't struggle. Always do what makes you feel comfortable. In this meditation, you are not trying to see or judge your body as ugly or beautiful but to see it as it is.

In the meditation, you might be able to see the details of your body quite clearly, or you might see just a vague general image. Or you might see only some parts clearly and visualize the structure of other parts incorrectly. Having a clear image of the body makes healing more effective, but the most important aspect of scanning the body is not necessarily to see all the details of the body clearly but to instill in the mind a sense of being in close contact with the details and characteristics of the body.

If you have difficulty seeing the image of the body or of any part, just think about the presence of the parts of the body and connect with them simply by thinking and feeling that you are seeing them as they are.

Then at the end of the scanning session, generate the feeling "Yes, I have seen or am seeing the whole body in detail, as it is," even if you are only seeing parts of it. For example, if you were watching a football game in a stadium, though you might be seeing only a few people in detail or clearly, or seeing just the faces and clothes of a few people, you might be able to think, feel, and believe that you were vividly seeing thousands of people. If you were looking at a good friend, you might not know everything about him or her, but you could think and feel, "I am seeing and knowing my friend completely."

So it is important to generate a feeling that "Yes, I have seen everything" when you are completing the scanning of your whole body. And even earlier, with each body part that you scan, it would be good to say to yourself and to feel, "Yes, I have seen this." This kind of recognition is a very good way of confirming and deepening the process. From this stage of meditation onward, take every opportunity to exercise the healing powers in

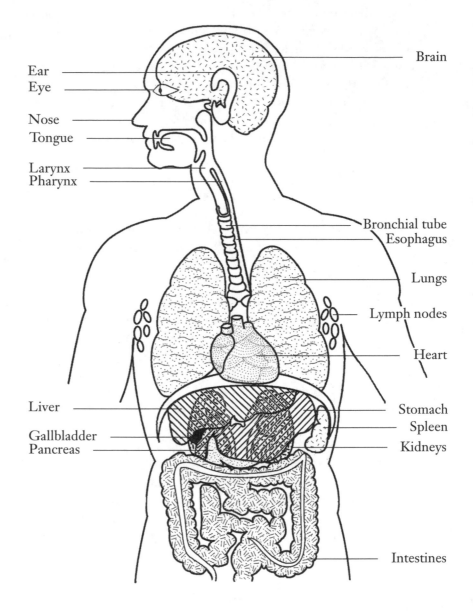

Ear

Eye

Nose

Tongue

Larynx

Pharynx

Brain

Bronchial tube

Esophagus

Lungs

Lymph nodes

Heart

Liver

Stomach

Spleen

Gallbladder

Pancreas

Kidneys

Intestines

this way: "I have seen everything," or "I am experiencing it all." This opens mind and body to healing.

In a later stage of the meditations, you will be using your mind to bring healing energies to your body. As much as possible, healing energies should be felt not only in the skin, muscles, and arteries but also in the organs and bones—throughout the body. This is how to bring healing from the mind to the body. However, I should also remind you that you should never grasp at healing images and feelings with attachment or craving. In meditation, whether you are scanning the body or calling forth healing energies, be relaxed and open. You connect to your body by scanning, and then you blossom openly with healing energies. Do this with a sense of freedom and relaxation, not tightness or grasping.

If you are someone whose body has any physical damage and you are ready to see it as it is, then seeing it will be beneficial to the healing process. But if seeing it would be disturbing, then just see the general image of the body without getting into the specific manifestations of that problem.

Perhaps you have not yet adapted to a change in your body produced by illness. In this case, you can see your body as it used to be before the illness. The goal is to establish a connection between body and mind but not necessarily with any particular form of the body.

Purpose: This meditation brings you into closer contact with your body. When your mind is connected intimately to your body, healing can permeate you. You have an open channel for positive energy. The healing you call upon in the other meditations on the body will become stronger and more powerful.

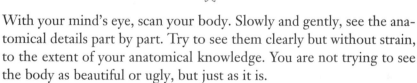

With your mind's eye, scan your body. Slowly and gently, see the anatomical details part by part. Try to see them clearly but without strain, to the extent of your anatomical knowledge. You are not trying to see the body as beautiful or ugly, but just as it is.

Relax and feel serenity in your body. You will be contemplating the body from head to feet.

First, with your mind's eye, scan the details of your head. See that your head is made of a skull and brain.

The Guided Meditations

See the sense organs: the eyes with their pupils, through which you see forms; the nose with its nostrils, through which you smell odors; the ears with their ear canals, through which you hear sounds; the tongue, with which you taste food; the teeth and jaws; the mouth, which enables you to eat and speak. See the facial muscles, the nerves and arteries, all the parts of the head covered with skin and hair. See your whole head as it is.

Now, with your mind's eye, scan your neck: see your throat, then the larynx and vocal cords, then the esophagus, leading into the stomach; also see the trachea, through which you breathe. See the skin covering it all.

Now scan your upper body: see the spine and spinal cord, the clavicle (collarbone), shoulder blades, sternum, and rib cage.

Scan the windpipe, which leads to the lungs, and see the soft, spongy lung tissue, which oxygenates the blood and removes carbon dioxide.

See the heart, which pumps blood through your body with its system of arteries.

Bring a sense of awareness to the nerves and vessels of this part of the body, the flesh and blood, all covered with skin.

Now scan your arms and hands: See the bones of the upper arms, forearms, hands, and fingers as well as the marrow within them. See the muscles, nerves, and blood vessels with blood coursing through them, all covered with skin.

Scan the internal organs and bones in the area of your abdomen. If you can't visualize all the details, focus mostly on major parts, such as your backbone, the pelvic bones, the stomach, kidneys, and intestines.

A more detailed picture would include: your spine and spinal cord; the pelvic bones; the liver on the right, with the gallbladder beneath it, the stomach to the left, the spleen farther to the left, the pancreas in the middle, the loops of small intestine, and the large intestine going up, across, then down on the left; the kidneys, which filter the blood; and the adrenal glands (located atop the large intestine), with their regulatory functions.

Bring your awareness to the urinary bladder, then to the male or female parts: either the ovaries and uterus or the prostate gland, and the genitalia.

See the nerves and vessels of this part of the body. See the muscles and connective tissue all covered with skin.

Scan your legs and feet: See the femurs (thighbones), tibias and fibulas (lower leg bones), and the bones of the feet and toes, with their bone marrow. See the muscles, nerves, and blood vessels of your legs and feet, all covered with skin.

Scan your lymph nodes, which are part of the immune system and are clustered at such strategic points as the neck, the armpits, and the groin.

Now look at your whole body. Your body is made of bones, organs, and muscles and has separate circulatory systems for blood and lymph fluid. All the bodily structures and organs and various fluids are wrapped in skin with tiny pores and hair.

The heart is pumping blood through every part of the body, blood that circulates through thousands of arteries and veins, carrying oxygen and nutrients and getting rid of waste. The lymph system with its vessels also permeates the body, producing disease-fighting lymphocytes, which are filtered in the lymph nodes.

Your exceedingly complex body parts are vibrantly functioning as one organism because of the circulating energy carried by the breath. As you breathe, feel your life's breath flowing through the body.

Think and feel that you have seen all the details of your body, just as they are. Think and feel that you have seen your whole body, just as it is.

Finally, enjoy the awareness of the vivid details of your body, your whole body, just as it is. Feel serenity, ease, and comfort in the vivid awareness of the body.

3.   *See Your Body as Made of Infinite Individual Cells*

Cells are the building blocks of the body. Having various shapes and colors, they are surrounded by a cell wall (membrane) filled with fluid (cytoplasm). As you can see in the accompanying illustration, they contain a nucleus and various vital structures within.

In Buddhist or Tibetan medical texts, I haven't found the concept of cells. Buddhism describes physical forms as collections of particles. Each particle is a composite of five elements: earth, water, fire, air, and space. However, instead of the image of particles, I chose the image of cells for the healing meditations, since they are more vivid and appealing for Westerners. Cells, after all,

81

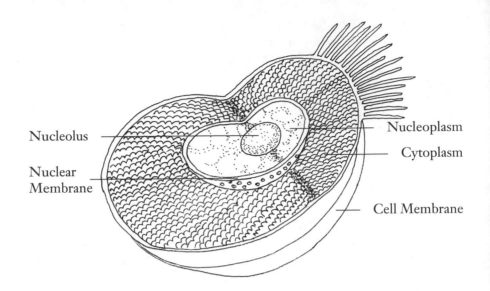

Nucleolus

Nuclear
Membrane

Nucleoplasm

Cytoplasm

Cell Membrane

are particles. If you prefer, you could think of the atoms in your body instead of cells. Or you could visualize particles and think of each particle as made of earth, water, fire, and air and functioning in space.

In this meditation, you will be visualizing the infinite quality of your body. Really allow your imagination to expand to take in the amazingly vast numbers of cells. If, at first, you have difficulty seeing clearly, you might begin with one or two cells, then a few, then many. Finally, *feel* as though you were clearly seeing very many cells, hundreds and even billions of them. The important point here is to develop, in a relaxed way, a strong feeling for the wondrous universe of cells within your body.

Purpose: This meditation creates a sense of seeing and feeling your body as a whole. Experiencing the infinite quality of your body opens up and eases the narrowness of your mind. The expansive mind is better able to approach the body. You begin to experience and appreciate the body's amazing structure.

This exercise and the previous one bring the mind and body in touch with each other directly and intimately. You are reconnecting to your body and making friends with it, and this helps all the different parts of your body, including your cells, to make friends with one another.

Healing Meditations on the Body

Your body is not just made of bones, flesh, and organs wrapped in skin. It is composed of trillions of cells.

Each part of your body is made of billions and billions of cells, individual cells. Cells are the building blocks of your body. They have all kinds of shapes, colors, and qualities. Most cells are a unit surrounded by a cell wall filled with fluid, holding various structures inside them.

Visualize in whatever way allows your mind to feel as if it is in touch with this vast array of cells. To make the interior of each cell more vivid and vital, you can see and think of each cell as having the qualities of earth, water, fire, and air. These qualities dwell in the open interior space of each cell.

With your mind's eye, see the cells of your body, part by part, slowly and gently, beginning with your head. Gradually move on to your upper body, arms and hands, abdomen, and legs and feet.

As your visualization progresses, think of one or two cells, then imagine that you are seeing a vast number of cells, even billions. Feel and believe that you are seeing a sweeping view of the infinite cells making up the parts of your body.

Feel that you are not fabricating this view, that your mind is touching the infinite cells, in their many different and individual shapes, colors, and designs.

First, see that your head is made of billions and billions of cells, individual cells with various designs, colors, and structures.

Then consider your upper body. See that it, too, is made of billions of individual cells, with all kinds of shapes, hues, and qualities.

See that your arms and hands are made of billions of cells, individual cells having many designs, colors, and functions.

See the billions of individual cells in your abdomen, with their variety of forms, shades, and structures.

And finally, see that your legs and feet are made of billions of cells, individual cells with all kinds of designs, colors, and qualities.

Now see and feel the infinite nature of the body. Your body is a collection of trillions of individual and distinctive cells, like a statue made of trillions of grains with various shapes, colors, and qualities.

Finally, rest in the feeling of the infinite nature of the body, without grasping at it or analyzing it.

Note: When you have gained some experience in this exercise and the others that follow, you may not need to meditate by going through the body part by part, from head to feet, in every session of meditation.

4. See Each Cell as a Cell of Light

By imagining that each cell in your body is illuminated with radiant light, you will be calling forth a particularly vital healing energy. Many spiritual traditions see light as associated with purity, freedom, holiness, or divinity. But you need not be a religious person to sense the powerful potential of light. Light makes the plants of the earth grow, and a sunny morning can make you feel good simply by its glorious radiance.

In Buddhism, meditations using light are considered an especially effective means of releasing the grasping qualities of tight minds, and this is the basis of all healing. Tibetans know about the healing energy of light firsthand, because visualizing light has been used effectively for many centuries to ease mental problems and suffering as well as physical sickness.

You can visualize light in three alternative ways, according to your needs and preferences:

1. See light without being restricted to visualizing a particular color; in other words, the light could be clear or white.
2. See light as multiple colors, like a rainbow.
3. See light as a particular color, such as red for warmth, blue for openness, or yellow for strength.

Although this book is about everyday healing, it might be helpful as background to describe in simplified terms how light is viewed in the ancient Tantric sources of Nyingma Buddhism, which I practice. According to the esoteric scriptures, mind and matter in their true nature are the inseparable union of wisdom and light. All matter is light. This is the enlightened view.

However, the ordinary, grasping mind sees reality not as the "oneness" of light but rather in the dualistic terms of subject and object. Because of these mental tendencies, our wisdom has become distilled into concepts and afflicting emotions, and the intangible, boundless radiance of wisdom light has been diminished to the gross elements.

The gross elements are earth, water, air, and fire, with the fifth being space. Each particle of the body is made of these five elements, which are manifested in different colors. In their true quality, space is blue light, water is white, earth is yellow, fire is red, and air is green.

I couldn't find any common (sutric) Buddhist source that describes matter in its true quality as light. However, I find it interesting that Western physics says that matter is actually energy, which can be manifested as light. Albert Einstein writes, "Mass and energy are therefore essentially alike; they are only different expressions for the same thing."[1]

So for scientists, the concept of matter, energy, and light as different expressions of the same thing is common knowledge. For Tibetan Buddhists, the highest understanding of matter is that it is light. Knowing all this may inspire you and help free up your meditation, since it implies that by contemplating light, you are touching the essential quality of nature and existence.

On the other hand, you don't need to be concerned with any of this in order to benefit from visualizing light. Just think of the beautiful, radiant, liberating quality of light. Doing so is relaxing and can bring well-being to both mind and body.

Purpose: Seeing yourself as a body of light can help you to feel clarity, peace, and joy. As light is pure, clear, luminous, and insubstantial, it does not lend itself to grasping and tightness. Visualizing light can be a very effective release from mental tensions, worries, sadness, and pain, which produce physical and mental rigidity and decay.

Seeing the body as light is a skillful means for developing a joyful disposition. Based on profound principles, this healing method helps ease your temporal problems and can lead you to higher spiritual realization.

The Guided Meditations

With your mind's eye, see once again that your body is made of billions of cells. Now visualize that these cells are cells of light. See this light as shining with different colors, like a rainbow. Feel as though radiant light were blossoming in each cell and throughout your body, bringing health and healing to each cell.

Slowly visualize light in every part of your body and even in all the cells within each part. See the cells of light as colorful, bright, translucent, insubstantial, and radiant.

Begin with your head. See the billions of cells of light there. Each one is a cell of bright, colorful, radiant light. The light shines and blossoms with health and healing.

See that your upper body is made of billions of individual cells of light, healing light that is bright, colorful, and radiant.

Focus on your arms and hands. See that they are also blossoming and shining with bright, colorful, radiant light.

See that your abdomen is radiant with wonderful healing light, bright and colorful.

Then see your legs and feet, with their billions of cells of light, each of which is bright, colorful, and radiant.

Now look at your whole body. Your body is composed of trillions of amazingly bright and colorful individual cells, like a bottle filled with grains of various shapes, colors, and qualities. All the cells of your body are radiant with bright, translucent, intangible light. Feel that healing light is shining forth throughout your body. This luminous display is taking place in billions of cells within your infinite body and shining or blossoming forth like flowers.

Bring your awareness to the insubstantial quality of light, which heals without limits, restrictions, or pressures. Enjoy the feeling of having a body of light. Relax in this feeling of freedom and peacefulness, without grasping at it or analyzing it.

5. *See Each Cell as Vast as the Universe*

With your imagination, you are going to choose one cell among the infinite cells of your body. Then you will enter into this cell and see and feel it as vast as the universe, boundless as space, peaceful, and filled with light as colorful as a rainbow.

Healing Meditations on the Body

The limitations of time and space are mere concepts created by the mind, designations of your own mind. In their true quality, according to Buddhism, time is timeless and space is boundless. When you see and feel the boundlessness of the space of a cell, your mind, too, opens boundlessly.

A story about the great Tibetan adept Milarepa illustrates the limitless nature of space. Milarepa was on a journey with his disciple Rechungpa, whose mind at that time was restricted and stained by his own arrogance. As they passed through an open field, they were beaten down by a heavy hailstorm. When the storm had somewhat calmed, Rechungpa couldn't find his teacher anywhere. But he heard Milarepa's singing voice coming from a dead yak's horn lying at a distance down the road.

Rechungpa tried to pick up the horn, but it was so heavy he couldn't move it. So, on hands and knees, he peered into the horn. There was Milarepa, singing his yogic songs with great joy, but his teacher didn't look any smaller and the horn didn't look any bigger. Milarepa spoke to his disciple: "If you are equal to me, son, just come in!" Rechungpa tried with all his might to climb inside but could not even force his fist in. At that point, all Rechungpa's arrogance vanished, and his spiritual path became effortless.

Like Rechungpa, you can become locked in a restrictive mindset. Being too forceful doesn't help. Instead, the right approach is to see that your mind is a vast resource that you may not have fully appreciated or used. You must be willing to cultivate the power of mind, gently and with devotion. To encourage these inner resources, you can use your imaginative powers in meditation. Your best allies are the four healing powers: thinking, recognizing, feeling, and believing. By seeing the boundless nature of your body, even down to its very cells, you are opening up your restricted mind and putting yourself on a positive path.

Purpose: Seeing and feeling the boundlessness of the cells in your body helps to release stress and pressure and to expand the scope of healing power and energies.

❀

With your mind's eye, visualize one particular cell in your body. A good place to begin is at your forehead, between your eyebrows. Or

The Guided Meditations

choose a cell from anywhere you feel is easy for you. Enter into that cell, as if you were entering a room.

See and feel that this cell is vast. It is as if you had entered outer space. Feel the boundless quality of this one cell and enjoy the amazing, radiant light that fills it, like a rainbow.

Use your imagination to move around the cell, to enjoy its vastness and beauty. This cell is calm and peaceful, like the clear and open sky. It is vast as the universe, boundless and calm, filled with lovely colors and light.

You could also see the cell as a vast, joyful world of fields, mountains, rivers, and gardens radiant with light and color.

Then go from this cell to ten neighboring cells. Look into each of them and, one after another, explore their variety. See rainbow light and feel boundless, skylike space or any other positive scenes. Use your imagination in a way that helps you appreciate the vastness and beauty.

Then expand your visualization so that you feel as though you were surveying the thousands or even billions of cells in the area of your forehead. Each one is boundless, radiant, and calm like the open sky.

You can then repeat this process of seeing the vastness of each cell in every part of your body—your head, upper body, arms and hands, abdomen, legs and feet. At each place, choose a cell and enter into it, as if you were entering a room.

Take your time seeing and feeling the vastness of this one cell. This cell is peaceful and clear like the open sky. It is as vast as the universe, boundless and calm, and radiant with lovely colors and light.

Move about in the neighboring cells, one after another, exploring their variety. Use your imagination to feel their wondrous vastness and peacefulness: see glorious rainbow light and feel the boundless, skylike space or see and feel any other lovely, positive scene. Expand your visualization so you feel that you are surveying the countless other cells in this part of your body. Each cell is boundless, radiant, and calm like the open sky.

Then survey your whole body, with its billions of vast, light-filled cells, and feel again the calmness like the clear, open sky. Feel that all the cells are in harmony with one another and that they are all sharing healing love.

Believe that you are not fabricating a vast, peaceful body but that

88

you are seeing its vastness just as is. Relax in this feeling, without grasping at it or analyzing it.

6. *Feel That Each Cell Is Filled with Healing Energies*

In this exercise, you will be calling on your inner resources to suffuse your body with the healing energies. You have already seen in your mind's eye the healing energy of light that illuminates each cell. Now you are going to bring other healing energies to these light-filled cells: heat and bliss.

Bringing healing energies to your body is at the heart of these exercises. So take your time and bask in the sense of well-being that this stage of the meditations gives you. The goal is to really feel that you are able to fill your whole being with warmth and joy, in every part and every cell of your body. Remember that your mind is amazing in its ability to heal. Let's say you are unsure of yourself as a beginner at meditation, or maybe you are a little skeptical and wonder, "How can I bring heat or bliss to the tiny cells in my body?" None of this matters, just so that for the duration of the meditation, you tell yourself you really see and believe and feel. If you are not quite sure what *bliss* is or don't like that term, use whatever positive words make you comfortable, as in, "My whole body, including all my cells, feels a wonderful sense of peace and happiness," or "I feel a healthy, healing warmth everywhere, in each and every cell of my body." Then notice whatever positive feelings you have and be happy about them.

Most people's health problems, especially in middle or old age, are caused by and manifested in the characteristics of coldness and sadness. So using the healing energies of heat and bliss is very beneficial.

Also note that it always helps, if you have trouble seeing many cells or particles, to focus your mind on one and then, if possible, expand the feeling to many.

While heat is the healing energy that most people will probably want to use, you could choose the essential quality of any particular element—earth, water, fire, air, or space—depending on your needs and what feels right. For example, instead of the heat of fire, use the quenching coolness of water for a fever; or

89

meditate upon the lightness of air or the openness of space if you have an enclosed or suffocating mentality; or see and feel that each cell has the stability of the earth if you are bothered by a floating sensation or a giddy mind.

Do this exercise with a sense of relaxation and comfort but also with enough dedication to allow your body to be immersed in the purifying energies of heat and bliss. If you prepare the way with this exercise, the meditation on healing waves that follows will be more effective.

Also, if you have proliferating cancer cells, it is an especially good idea to take your time immersing yourself in the purifying healing energies. This avoids any risk of mental negativity or physical toxins being spread instead of transformed when you begin the healing waves.

Purpose: Developing an awareness of healing energies is one of the most vital exercises in these meditations. You are planting the seeds to purify the ills of mind and body. By imagining the positive transformation of infinite cells, you are gaining practice in boundless joy. As you work with this meditation, you can learn how to melt away cold and sadness. You can awaken a feeling of enjoyment and peace in your life that you didn't think possible. This is a powerful meditation to promote well-being.

❁

Again with your mind's eye, look at your forehead, between the eyebrows, and choose one cell of light to enter from among the billions of cells.

In your imagination, go into this vast cell, as if entering a room. Now move around in it and feel that the cell is not just vast like outer space but that it is filled with the healing energies of heat and bliss or, if you prefer, warmth and joy.

Use your imagination to really feel that this is a very happy place, with no cold or pain, only warmth and total contentment. The cell is filled with blissful warmth, with no pressure, only comfort. It is a spacious, open cell, like the clear sky. It is filled to capacity with light and warmth and is a delightful place to be, like coming into a perfectly heated or warmed room in winter. Bask in the healing energy filling this boundless cell.

Now see that your forehead is a collection of hundreds of thousands of individual cells and recognize that every one of them is a boundless cell of light. Each one is filled to capacity with the healing energy of heat and bliss.

In your mind's eye, you can visit each part of your body, seeing and feeling that each of the countless individual cells of light is vast. Feel that all of them are filled completely with the healing energies of heat and bliss.

Bask in the wonderful feeling of blissful heat in every spacious cell of all the parts of your body. Take your time at each part: your head, upper body, arms and hands, abdomen, and legs and feet.

If any part or parts of your body need special healing, spend more time there. Bringing your attention to the area, see the billions of individual cells, cells of light. Feel that each cell is filled to capacity with the healing energy of blissful heat.

Bring your awareness to your whole body, with its trillions of individual cells. See that each cell of your body is a boundless cell of light. Feel that each cell is filled with the healing energy of blissful heat. Bask in that delightful feeling. Really feel that your whole body is totally filled with bliss, heat, and comfort.

Then think and feel that the cells of your body are not just filled with healing energies but that they are also generating powerful healing energies. Feel that the power of blissful heat has completely purified all your mental impurities and eliminated the physical toxins from every cell of your body, leaving no trace. Focus your awareness and belief on this feeling of total purity in every cell of your body.

Finally, enjoy the feeling of your body as a body of infinite, boundless, and pure healing energies. Relax in open awareness of the healing energies, the blissful heat of your body, in total silence, without grasping or analyzing.

7.   *Heal Your Body with Waves of Light and Energy*

You can enhance the power of the healing energies by using your breathing as the benevolent force that acts like a purifying wind. In this guided meditation, you'll use your breathing to send healing waves through your body. As you exhale and inhale, you will think and feel that light and especially heat and bliss are carried

The Guided Meditations

to every cell of your body. This is the main meditation to heal the ills of mind and body.

In the workshops that I have led, it's no wonder that people seem to respond to this exercise with tremendous enjoyment and enthusiasm. This is a very active meditation, and it employs the breath, which is, after all, the wellspring of life. When you synchronize your breathing with positive energy, the results can be quite potent.

Although the healing energy is carried upon powerful waves, the flow should be natural, easy, and open. You should not be too forceful, because this can tighten you up and turn the energy negative. If you find yourself being too aggressive, or feel constriction or giddiness, try to relax. Go back to a simple contemplation of your breathing and relax your abdomen as you breathe, so that the stomach gently and naturally rises with each inhalation. You might think of your breathing as a gentle wind that is soothing and calm.

If you have any particular problem—your stomach is knotted with anxiety, let's say—first determine where that problem is located and visualize it in whatever form seems appropriate to you. You could see the problem as a knot or as darkness or as ice. If your problem is a wound, an inflammation, or a feverish swelling, perhaps see it as a flame. Then bring healing waves to that part of the body, visualizing the cells there if possible. Heat and bliss are the common forms of energy, but if your problem takes the form of a flame, you will want to visualize images that cool or melt, such as healing water.

If you are sick and taking medicine or receiving some other treatment, you can coordinate, or harmonize, the meditation of healing waves with the treatment. That way, as the medicine enters and is absorbed into your body, the benefit will be maximized.

Purpose: This stage of the meditations awakens and invigorates the healing of every part of the body and every aspect of the mind. The movement of waves unites the body in generating and sharing healing energy. The aim of the healing waves is to clear blockages, reconnect or repair damage, and bring life and health back to sick cells.

As you become familiar with the movements of the healing

Healing Meditations on the Body

waves and practice generating them, it will become easier for your nervous system to live in harmony with the rest of your body and for you to be healthier and happier.

※

Bring your awareness to the breath in your body. Relax your stomach and allow the breathing to be natural and unforced. Be aware of your breathing in and breathing out, as your breath comes up from the abdomen and fills your respiratory system.

As your breath is moving through your body, think and feel that all the cells of your body are also breathing. All the trillions of cells of light and blissful heat are breathing, from the top of your head to the soles of your feet. Your breath is moving through your whole body, and all the cells in your body are exhaling and inhaling continuously.

Now feel that the breathing is the movement not just of air but of powerful waves of healing light and healing energy. Your very breathing is heat and bliss. Your very breathing moves through your body as waves of powerful healing energy.

Every cell in your body is overflowing with healing energy, and the waves of blissful heat are strengthening and redoubling the healing power as they move through your body.

As you exhale, think and feel that all the cells of your body are sending out waves of healing energy, blissful heat, as offerings to all the other cells of your body, from the top of your head to the soles of your feet.

As you inhale, think and feel that all the cells of your body are taking in waves of healing energy, blissful heat, as gifts from all the other cells of your body, from the top of your head to the soles of your feet.

Think and feel that all the cells of your whole body are participating as one team in sending and receiving gifts of healing energy waves, waves of blissful heat. Feel the waves of healing energy, blissful heat.

Think and feel that all the cells are interconnected by the current of energy waves moving through your body, the waves of blissful heat. All the cells are actively sending and receiving energy waves as one team. As the waves of energy move, the healing energy, blissful heat, increases in every cell of your body and in your body as a whole.

See and feel the amazing stimulation of healing energy. The waves surge from every part of your body and infuse every part of your body,

93

filling every boundless cell of your body. Enjoy these amazing waves of healing energy as they move up and down, in and out, of each of your body's boundless cells of light. Everywhere in your body, every single cell is totally filled by these amazing, surging healing waves.

Now see, feel, and believe that all sick and dying cells in your body are brought back to life, with the nourishing waves of healing light and energy, as water revives a wilted flower.

See, feel, and believe that these wonderful, powerful waves have brought healing and health to all of your body: feel that hardened arteries have become elastic; feel that any and all of the blockages in the arteries have been cleared by the power of the waves of healing light and energy; feel that any and all broken or weakened tissues or internal parts have been repaired and reconnected. Your whole body is functioning as one, linked by the healing of these powerful waves.

As the rhythm of your breathing sends healing waves through your body, see and feel that the coldness and sadness of your mind and body are melted in a stream of joyful light and blissful heat.

See, feel, and believe that your whole body and mind is blossoming with joy, comfort, peace, and well-being because of the waves of blissful heat surging through your body.

Again and again, bring your awareness to your body and its collection of billions and billions of cells of light. The healing waves flow like a current through every cell, connecting them together. Enjoy the feeling in your body as the healing waves move through it. Enjoy the feeling that your body is a body of healing energy, amazing health, and well-being.

When you feel complete in this meditation, relax in a state of open awareness and silence. Be one with whatever you are experiencing, like water being poured into water.

Note: A number of alternative ways of practicing this exercise could be useful:

- If, in the beginning, you feel too rushed sending and receiving the healing waves with every breath, then first, for many cycles of breathing, focus on your exhalation, sending out healing waves of light and blissful heat. The outgoing breath becomes the waves, sending healing to the cells of your body.

  Then, for many cycles of breathing, focus on your inhalation, which brings healing light and the energy of blissful heat to all your cells. As you inhale, every cell of your body receives the gift of healing from every other cell in your body.

Then, when you feel comfortable, return to the meditation of sending and receiving healing energy waves with every inhalation and exhalation.

- When exhaling, think and feel that the cells of your body are creating a cloud of healing light and energy in your body, as a greenhouse is filled with the scents of flowers or the atmosphere is filled with the warmth of sunlight.

When inhaling, think and feel that each cell is receiving waves of healing light and energy from the reservoir created by this healing cloud.

- If this meditation is aimed at healing a particular mental or physical problem, do the following: Briefly see and feel your particular problem in the form of an appropriate image, such as ice or darkness, at the location where you experience it most strongly. Then see and feel that the healing waves are totally healing your problem and enjoy the relief from that problem.

- If this meditation produces uneasy sensations or makes you feel too high, floaty, or jumpy, you may simply need to relax and ease back a bit. Try focusing less on the power and movement of the healing waves. Instead, emphasize a more relaxed, open awareness of soothing warmth and healing.

Or do an appropriate exercise, such as "Dispelling Uneasy Sensations" or "Grounding the Floating Mind," described in stage 1 of these meditations.

Perform a Special Meditation to Heal Proliferating Sick Cells (Optional)

Some people are concerned that if you have a proliferating sickness such as cancer, then you shouldn't use energy waves, as they might cause the cancer to metastasize rather than healing it.

I disagree. If you do this meditation properly, with a relaxed and positive mind, it will bring beneficial results.

However, if you have misgivings about energy waves' causing the cancer to spread, the power of your mind's fear could erode the meditation and even pose a risk. So if you have cancer or a proliferating sickness and are concerned about making the problem worse, it might be better to do this special alternative meditation. This version of the exercise would also be beneficial for other ailments, such as stomach problems.

In the exercise, you will be imagining a wall of positive energy around the sick cells, which will contain them and allow healing to take place. You will also visualize the billions of healthy cells surrounding the sick area and see this healthy part of your body as radiating healing energy. So you have a defensive shell that limits the cancer and an offensive force that overwhelms it with healing.

Alternatively, in the seventh, eighth, and ninth stages, you could meditate in the following way, especially if the cancer has spread into many parts of your body: See and feel that all the cells, including the sick cells, are boundless cells of light filled with healing energies. Each affected cell is burning its cancer by the force of its own healing energy and has turned into a cell of healing energies, as fire burns wood and turns it into flame.

Sickness can be such a difficult time. If your emotions are being buffeted by anxiety and sadness, you can use this meditation as a refuge. Make up your mind that during the meditation, you will feel comfort and peace. This can be a time of great soothing, when you care for yourself, without worries. You should visualize as clearly as possible and feel the power of the healing energies. Linger on the image of the healthy cells surrounding your sick cells and on the healing that is radiating from them to the cancerous cells or tumor.

You could see your body as it now appears—with any changes in form, color, or structure that might have occurred due to sickness. Then see that those changes are healed and that you have resumed the form of your original healthy self.

Finally, you can expand your meditation by wishing health and peace for everyone else in the world. When you are sick, it can be very beneficial for your well-being to feel compassion for others. It gets you out of yourself and allows you to transform your own suffering into something positive. In the process of being compassionate, your mind and body are spontaneously energized with positive energy, which, in turn, can be a source of healing for you.

Purpose: Not every sickness can be cured. Even the Buddha grew old, became ill, and died. However, your body has tremendous natural resources for healing, and you can encourage your bodily defenses, even as you can be helped by medicines and doctors. This meditation is only one of many that are beneficial for cancer or proliferating sickness. For example, you could visualize healing nectar or healing energy using specifically Buddhist imagery, as described in Part Three.

❊

If you know that you have any cancerous, proliferating sick cells, then visualize those cells in their present structure, color, and feeling, at their location, according to what you know and however much it is easy for you.

Bring your awareness as best you can to the unaffected parts of your body and recognize the cells there as strong and healthy. Each cell is as vast as the universe. Each is a cell of healing light and healing energy: heat and bliss, powerful, blissful heat.

Meditate again and again on the healthy cells that surround the sick cells. See and feel the healthy cells as pure and radiant with light. In particular, feel the amazing positive force of blissful hot energy from these healthy cells.

Now see and feel that a powerful wall of energy is formed around the sick cells, like an eggshell. No negative energy can penetrate this wall and feed or nourish the sick cells, and no harmful energy from the sick cells can escape through the wall to damage other cells. The sick cells are totally isolated, disconnected, and starved to death.

As you exhale and inhale, feel that every healthy cell of your body is also breathing. As you breathe, waves of healing energy from every healthy cell of your body are aimed at the sick area. Feel and enjoy the power of the blissful heat coming from the healthy cells of your body.

As you breathe, every healthy cell of your upper body is sending down waves of light and blissfully hot energy toward the sick cells. As you breathe, every healthy cell of your lower body is sending up waves of blissfully hot energy toward the sick cells.

Now, as you breathe, think and feel that the waves of blissful heat energy are touching the sick cells and that they are slowly starting to soften. Keep watching that image. Feel the experience of the sick cells softening and changing. The sick cells are gradually starting to melt.

The blissful heat waves melt the sick cells into liquid, first in a trickle, then in a flood of fluid. As you breathe, healing waves discharge the flood of melted sick cells through the two lower exits of your body. All the sick cells with their ills are completely purged. They leave your body and dissolve in air without leaving a trace. Bring your awareness to your body and feel that you are now totally free of sick cells and sickness. Enjoy the feeling of vacancy and freedom from illness in your body.

Repeat this exercise as many times as you comfortably can.

Then see and feel that your healthy cells are producing pure new cells, thousands and billions of them. These new healthy cells, filled with light and healing energy, are taking the place of the melted cells. Now your whole body is composed of beautiful, strong, healthy cells filled with amazing healing energy.

Enjoy the wonderful, powerful feeling of blissful heat and the feeling of freedom from sickness. Finally, relax in open awareness of your experience, without grasping at it or analyzing it.

8.   *Hear the Healing Sound of* AH

Chanting and singing are among the most powerful means of healing in many of the world's traditions and cultures. Any inspiring sound—such as a prayer, a mantra, a sacred name, a phrase, or a syllable—can be used for the sound of healing.

Here the sound AH is used. You say or sing AH while exhaling and hear the sound AH in your mind while inhaling. You could sing AH loudly or else just hear the sound in your mind, as you prefer. Simultaneously, you will be using the sound AH to generate and strengthen the healing waves as they move through your body.

According to the teachings of Buddhism, AH is the source and essence of all sound. All sounds, words, language, and prayer come out of AH. Further, AH is in all sounds, words, language, and prayer.

At the same time, AH does not contain or impose concepts, messages, or emotional afflictions. Rather, AH is the sound of boundless energy, openness, freedom, and peace. It is a natural sound endowed with releasing, opening, and healing qualities. Its quality is similar to space. Space provides the sphere within which all the phenomena can arise and function, but it does not impose structure or conditions.

In Tibetan Buddhist scriptures, AH is the essence of all the teachings on transcendental wisdom (*prajnaparamita*). It is the unborn and uncreated letter, the letter of openness or emptiness, the great mother of all.

You don't have to be Buddhist, or even religious, to appreciate the sound AH. It has a warm, soothing, open-throated quality as you say or sing it. So as you do this meditation, enjoy this sound. To get the full benefit of this exercise, relax your stomach as you breathe in. Then, as you sing AH, the breath can fully come up from the diaphragm. The sound AH is the sound of your breathing. It is the sound of the healing waves moving through your body.

Purpose: The sound AH reinforces the healing energies in your body and mind. It intensifies the power of the energy waves and helps to release you from the bondage of physical and mental afflictions.

Bring awareness to your breathing. Meditate once again upon the waves of healing energy and light, moving in and out of every cell of your body in sync with your breathing.

Now add the soothing sound AH, the sound of openness, freedom, and peace. It is also the sound of healing in the form of the waves of blissful heat. The healing waves are blossoming with the sound AH, as they move in and out on your breath.

Sing AH in three tones of voice:

1. In a loud and inspiring voice, sing AH, the sound of healing light and blissful heat.

    While exhaling, think and feel that all the cells of your body, with love, are sending the offering of the singing sound of AH, the sound of healing, to all the other cells of your body, from the top of your head to the soles of your feet.

    While inhaling, just hear the singing sound of AH and feel that every cell of your body, from head to toe, is joyfully hearing the healing sound of AH.

    Exhaling, sing the sound AH, and inhaling, hear the singing sound of AH.

All the cells of your body, from the top of your head to the soles of your feet, are enjoying AH, the sound of healing waves of light and energy, like the joyous sound waves of a great symphony. Feel that the sound of AH is awakening all the cells and bringing boundless blissful heat and radiant light to each cell. With each AH, your mind and body blossom with health and healing.

2. In a soft voice, as if you were almost whispering, sing AH as you exhale. This soft, lovely sound sends waves of healing from every cell of your body to every other cell.

   While inhaling, just hear the soft, singing sound of AH. Feel that every cell of your body is joyfully receiving the sound of AH with its healing light and blissful heat.

3. In the silent voice of the mind, sing the sound AH. Silently sing AH as you exhale and inhale. Feel that every cell of your body, with love, is sending waves of healing to all the other cells and also receiving healing from all the other cells.

Every cell of your body, from the top of your head to the soles of your feet, is enjoying the singing sound of AH, the sound of the healing waves of light and blissful, soothing, healing heat.

Bring your awareness to AH and enjoy the sound as it brings healing energy to your mind and body. Then, in silence, rest in open awareness of what you are experiencing, without grasping.

Note: Here are some alternatives to this exercise:

- If you feel rushed or overly active when you focus on every exhalation and inhalation, try focusing for the first few breathing cycles only on the sound of AH being sent out. Then, for the next few breathing cycles, focus on the cells of your body receiving the healing sound.

   Or if you feel that you are being overwhelmed by the energy of the sound waves, focus for a while only on the waves being sent out.

- As you exhale, sing AH and feel that clouds of healing light and energy are filling your body, as the earth is filled with the warmth of sunlight. As you inhale, feel that each cell of your body is receiving the healing gift of AH, in the form of a vast reservoir of healing clouds.

9. *Open to Healing with the Blossoming Lotus Movement*

Physical movement—such as processions, dances, hand gestures, and hand blessings—is a fundamental part of ritual and healing

Healing Meditations on the Body

in many traditions. Every living thing is changing—growing, living, or decaying—through movement. Things connect and harmonize with one another through movement or disconnect and are destroyed. When healing energy is harnessed to movement, the positive results are maximized.

However, movement without awareness generates very little healing energy or none at all. In many cases, it only burns up your energy. So I would urge to you to really focus in this exercise on being aware, even when you are doing a very subtle movement.

Any number of movements can be used as a means of meditative healing. But here you will be using a simple hand gesture based on the unfolding of the lotus flower.

The lotus has especially positive spiritual associations. It grows in mud and slime, and yet its blossom is extraordinarily beautiful. This is like we are as ordinary humans, afflicted by sufferings and impurities and yet unstained and perfect in our true nature.

In this exercise, you'll join your hands together, fingertips touching and palms toward each other or touching. Then you will open your hands in a blossoming motion. Your awareness of the healing power of the movement should unfold very deliberately and slowly. And so, even before doing any physical movement, you should concentrate on your breathing and feel that your whole body, even every cell, is also breathing in and out.

At the beginning, you move very little, as if you were hardly moving at all, or as if the movement were almost mental rather than physical. Concentration is the key. Then, at every moment of this exercise, be totally aware.

The important thing is not necessarily to create any beautiful movement but to be fully aware of the movements at the most subtle level of energy. Be aware of the delightful feeling as your body, and even every cell, opens to the healing gesture.

When you touch your fingers and palms together, this movement should be synchronized with the mental feeling that the cells of your body are touching, connecting, and sharing healing energies with one another. When you open your fingers and palms, this movement should be done with the mental feeling that your cells are opening and blossoming.

In this exercise, it is also very powerful to coordinate the gesture with the movement of healing waves. You could also sing the

The Guided Meditations

sound AH with the movements. The combination of movement and sound intensifies the healing.

Purpose: Physical movements such as the lotus gesture maximize the healing energy. Movement activates your body so that every part can share in the healing. It strengthens the benefits to body and mind. The movement speeds up healing in the body and helps to liberate your mind from mental and emotional restrictions.

Movement with awareness can generate amazing healing energies. If you are aware of the healing energies as you move, and if you add the healing power of sound, the benefits to mind and body can be intensified, just as a fire is intensified when fanned by wind.

❦

Fold your hands together at your heart in the shape of a flower bud, with palms toward or touching each other and the tips of your fingers lightly touching (see the accompanying illustration). Bring your awareness, with total attention, to the touch of your hands together. Spend some time in careful awareness of your breathing and of your fingertips or hands touching.

Be aware, during this meditation, that your relaxed breathing is generating healing waves, which permeate your body and all your boundless cells. Feel that the healing movements are redoubling the power of blissful heat energy.

Think of your fingers and hands as being made of billions of cells of light. Each cell is vast and overflowing with healing energy. Every cell is sending blissful healing waves to every other cell and receiving them from every other cell.

With total awareness, think and feel that all the cells of your fingers and hands are touching one another, as the petals and pistils of a flower bud are connected. Bring your total and undivided awareness to the feeling of connection.

Feel that the cells of your fingers and hands are connected by a chain of energy. Notice any feeling of connection, like a current of energy, and allow that feeling to blossom and grow. Think that if you move your fingers slightly, or move even one cell, you will notice a feeling of connection among the cells in your two hands, as if the cells in your hands were attached by an invisible string. Then expand your awareness to feel the connection of energy among all the cells of your fingers, hands, arms, and your whole body.

102

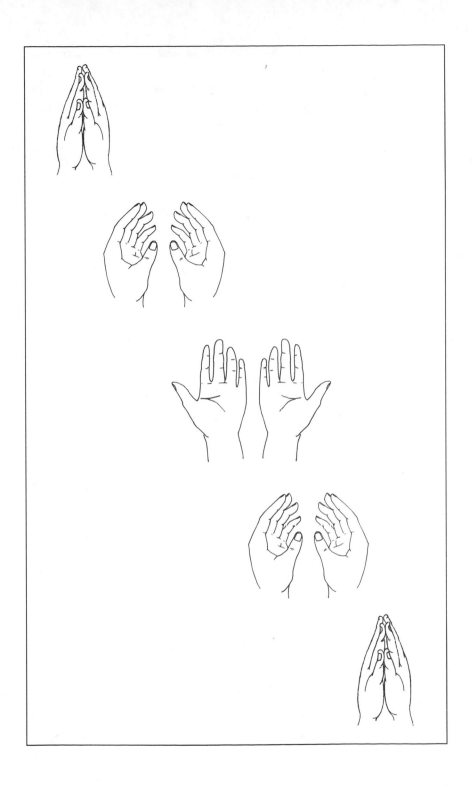

Feel that the healing energy of heat and bliss is making the connection stronger.

Now, open your palms in the form of a blossoming flower, in utmost slow motion, as if they were hardly moving. Slowly move your hands apart sideways until they are about six or eight inches apart, or as wide as feels comfortable to you.

While your hands are slowly opening, think of them as opening the way a flower opens and blossoms. Think, feel, and believe that this movement of your hands is activating waves of healing energy, blissful heat, throughout every cell of your fingers and hands, like the flow of a river. The movement is strengthening and redoubling the healing energy, like turning on a light switch or the handle of a water faucet.

Very slowly close your hands, like the petals of a flower closing, and feel that as you do, you are feeling the healing connection among all the cells in your hands.

Repeat the blossoming gesture of your hands, slowly opening, slowly closing. As you do so, bring your awareness to each part of your body. As you open, feel that you are activating or bringing healing energy to that part of the body. As you close, feel that all the cells in that part of the body are touching one another and sharing wonderful healing energy.

So very slowly open your hands and bring awareness to the current of healing energies blossoming in your arms. Very slowly close your hands and feel that every cell in both arms is touching and sharing the wonderful healing energy.

Again, slowly open your hands and feel that the gesture of opening is activating waves of healing energy like a current through all the cells of your upper body.

Then slowly close your hands and feel that all the cells in your upper body are joining and touching one another, like the petals of a flower bud. Feel that as the cells touch one another, they are sharing healing energy. Feel the energy flowing like a healing current through every cell.

Move on to your head, your abdomen, and then your legs and feet.

Slowly open your hands and feel that the gesture of opening is activating waves of healing energy in the area on which you are focusing.

Slowly close your hands and feel that all the cells in the area on which you are focusing are touching one another and sharing healing

Healing Meditations on the Body

energy, like the petals of a flower bud. Feel the energy flowing like a healing current through every cell.

Finally, perform the blossoming lotus gesture with the feeling that your whole body is involved in healing. As you open your hands, the healing energy blossoms in your body. As you close them, feel that every cell of your body is sharing the amazing, powerful, healing energies of heat, bliss, and light.

Repeat the gesture as many times as you like. As you open your hands, you are opening to healing. As you close your hands, you are bringing healing to every cell of your body.

You could also synchronize the singing sound of AH with the movements.

Enjoy the blissful heat of healing as it flows through your body. Then just relax in open awareness of the experience, silently.

Note: As your meditation progresses, you could also open to healing in the movements of your daily life. You can think and feel that you are generating a current of healing energy by such movements as standing and rocking from side to side, walking, slowly dancing, doing yoga exercises, or even running. All these movements could become the means of creating and harmonizing the healing energy current and flow of your body.

Open to Healing with Other Movements to Relieve Physical Ailments and Promote General Health (Optional)

Although the lotus gesture is a very good way to intensify the healing energies in the body, I have discovered from my own experience that a number of other physical movements can be even more effective in healing particular problems.

These movements are aimed at releasing stiffness, muscle and joint strains, blockages and pain, and congestion. While I have found the healing movements very useful when adapted to heal a particular ailment, they could also serve as a method of preventing problems before they arise as well as generally maintaining physical health.

I suffered from a lower-back problem for years. My chiropractor treated me horizontally on a table, holding my upper spine upward and pushing my lower spine downward to open my crushed lumbar vertebrae. But for the last couple of years, whenever my back has gone out, I have done stretching movements with healing energy waves on my own. They healed even the worst episodes in a couple of days.

First, I lay on my back on a floor mat and relaxed for a minute or two. Then I generated the feeling of healing energy and the energy waves in my body. When I felt I was being immersed in the healing energies, I very slowly began stretching my back. I pulled my upper body and spine upward, as if growing like a tree, while simultaneously pushing my lower body and spine downward, a motion at about the same energy level.

In addition to being aware of the energy waves throughout my whole body, I focused my awareness specifically on the feeling in the area of my crushed lumbar vertebrae. My mind generated the feeling and belief that the vertebrae were moving apart, releasing the disks, nerves, and cartilage with healing light, energy, and motion.

Then, following this stretching movement, I brought the same awareness to slowly relaxing my body and my back to their normal position. Each cycle of stretching and relaxing took about a minute or so. I repeated the movement for ten or fifteen minutes at a time, three or four times a day.

It is especially effective if you are able to diagnose the problem and know how to tailor a movement to remedy the ailment. In my case, a chiropractor had shown me the proper movement to remedy the particular back problem.

You could do the various healing movements sitting in a lotus posture or in a chair or else standing or lying down. The best position for several of the movements, especially the stretching, is to lie on your back in bed or on a mat on the floor. These exercises should be done, insofar as possible, in a peaceful setting in which the temperature is comfortable for you.

The exercises can be done as part of the twelve stages of healing meditation or on their own, depending on your level of experience. If you are fairly advanced, it may be possible in just a couple of minutes to relax your body and call up a general feeling of healing energy before starting the movements.

Healing Meditations on the Body

With any meditation, but especially these movement exercises, you should bring yourself back to awareness if you start to drift into distraction or a sleepy state of mind. These movements are very subtle, and much of the energy is generated on the mental level. So you need to really focus your awareness on the healing energies. If you do the movements very slowly and gradually, with total concentration, you hardly need to move at all to become aware of the energy in your body.

I like to compare the energy flow in the body to the movement of beads on a string. The goal is to feel and believe that you are generating positive energy that is being shared by the parts of your body. Your whole body is working together as a team, in a kind of chain reaction of energy, like beads moving in unison when the string is shifted.

The movements used in healing meditation share some similarities with movements that are done in conventional physical exercises or in therapies like massage. When you exercise a muscle, you exert the muscle and it tightens, then you relax the muscle and rest it. When you massage a muscle, you press or rub the muscle, then release it. In the healing meditations, you also close and then open, stretch or tighten and then relax. The big difference is that the movement is at a subtle energy level.

Although your awareness is focused, the feeling in your mind and body should remain relaxed and open, not tense or forced. One of the exercises calls for you to tighten your muscles slightly, but this shouldn't be done aggressively. If you feel excessive energy or tightness, relax and open up your feelings. In other words, your mind needs to let go of grasping as much as possible.

Purpose: Physical movement can intensify the healing energy of body and mind. Your mind and body become closely connected, with the mind generating a strong flow of healing energy. The blockages in your body are released and opened, which can maximize the healing of particular problems such as back strains. These healing movements are helpful for maintaining general health as well as relieving specific ailments.

❋

To intensify healing in muscles, joints, and other parts of your body, do any of the following physical movements or do all of them one after

The Guided Meditations

another. You can perform these movements in whatever position is comfortable, such as lying down or standing.

Before beginning any of these movements, establish contact with the healing energies of your body.

Immerse yourself in awareness of the healing energies in every boundless cell of light of your body. Bathe in the feeling of healing energies. Feel the movements of the waves of healing energies in your body and in every boundless cell of light of your body.

Stretching and Relaxing. Very slowly stretch your body, your joints and muscles, for a minute or so. Stretch the upper part of your body upward, like a tree growing up to the sky, and the lower part of your body downward, like roots reaching toward the earth. With total awareness, feel the energy being generated by the slow, subtle movement.

Feel that the movement is activating chain reactions of healing energy, blissful heat, throughout every cell of your body, like the flow of a river. Bring your awareness to any particular problem—for example, any injured or blocked area—and feel the flow of energy bringing the maximum amount of healing to all the boundless cells of this area. Continue this stretch for a minute or so or for however long is comfortable.

Then relax your body. Take about a minute to do this, allowing the joints and muscles to move back into place. Feel the blissful heat of the healing energy moving and flowing through your body as you do this. The positive energy is being absorbed in your body, healing any problem areas.

Slowly repeat the same stretching and relaxing of your body. Be aware of the feelings of your subtle movements, the stretching and relaxing of your body. Feel that every part of your body is sharing energy with every other part. Feel the interconnectedness of all the parts of your body. Feel the flow of energy, like a river or current, as all the boundless cells of your body work together as a team to heal your body and any problem areas.

Note: The movements in all these exercises should be done with very relaxed breathing. In whatever way you find comfortable, you could synchronize your inhalation and exhalation with the movements.

Note, also, that instead of the stretching movement, or in addition to it, you could lie on your back and do a very slow bicycle-pedaling

Healing Meditations on the Body

motion with your feet. As in the preceding exercise, the movements are very subtle. Your mind generates the feeling of an energy flow in sync with this subtle physical movement. Feel the flow of energy throughout your whole body and in all your boundless cells.

Expanding Your Body as You Breathe. With total awareness, very slowly expand your body as you inhale. Feel the relaxed expansion of your stomach as you inhale; feel your chest expand. Feel that as you inhale, your whole body is expanding—the organs, the muscles, the nerves. Feel that this movement is activating a wonderful flow of healing energy. Then relax your body as you exhale and feel that the muscles, organs, and nerves are relaxing back into place. Be aware of the subtle movements of expansion and relaxation of your body and every one of its cells. As in all these healing movements, you can focus your awareness on any particular problem and maximize the healing there.

Rejoice in the flow of healing energy, blissful heat, as your body opens to healing with these movements. Slowly repeat the expansion and relaxation of your body again and again.

Tightening and Relaxing. With total awareness, very slowly tighten the muscles of your body for a minute or so. Feel that this subtle tightening or contracting of muscles is activating the blissful heat energy. Feel and believe that all the boundless cells of your body are touching one another as your muscles gently contract. They are connecting with one another like a team and sharing the blissful flow of healing energy.

Then relax the muscles of your body for a minute or so. Feel the release of your muscles and joints. Feel that the flow of blissful heat energy is being absorbed as the boundless cells of your body open to healing.

The tightening and relaxing are so subtle that the movements may or may not even be visible but are felt at the energy level.

Slowly repeat the tightening and relaxing of the muscles of your body again and again, with total awareness of the subtle movements of tightening and relaxing.

Swaying Your Body. With total awareness, very slowly sway or rock your body and every cell of your body to one side and then the other (or backward and forward). The swaying is very, very subtle and slow, and the motion is very slight, even less than an inch in either direction. Feel that this gentle, subtle movement is activating powerful chain reactions of healing energy, which all your cells share. Feel that a flow of energy, like a current or river, is connecting all the boundless cells of your body. Sway to the right for a minute or so, then to the left for a minute or so. Slowly repeat the swaying again and again.

The swaying is so subtle that the movements may or may not be visible but are felt at the energy level.

When you feel complete with any of the preceding exercises, or at the end of them all, rejoice in any positive feeling. Finally, relax in oneness with the experience without grasping or needing to think or analyze.

10. *Share the Healing Waves with Others*

Up to this point, you have been concentrating on healing yourself, which is the proper thing to do. Healing yourself gives you the strength to be more selfless. Now, in this stage of the exercises, you enlarge your meditation to include others.

A core religious practice throughout the world is the sharing of blessings with others. In Tibetan Buddhism, meditation practice is always dedicated to helping other sentient beings. Even secular humanists believe that the impulse of wanting others to be well is one of humanity's noblest characteristics.

In this exercise, you will visualize that healing light and energy are flowing beyond you to heal others.

So first you focus on healing yourself, and that way you can gain strength to heal others. Of course, when this dedication is sincerely practiced, it has a secondary benefit: it loosens your grasping after your tight little self and your personal problems, widens the perspective of your place in the world, and can make you happier and less anxious.

Purpose: This selfless meditation helps you heal others, which is the whole point of the training. But if you meditate on healing others, you will in the process also maximize the power and speed with which your own problems are healed.

❧

Think and feel that your body is made of billions of boundless cells, cells of amazingly bright and colorful healing light. All the cells are filled with and are emitting waves of healing light and blissful heat energy. Your whole body is also filled with and sending outward the healing sound AH, with love.

Healing Meditations on the Body

Then, visualize a particular person or persons with whom you wish to share your healing power. See the people and their problems in accurate images to the extent that you can. Alternatively, you could send healing power to the people of a particular land or country.

Think and feel that from all the boundless cells of your body, beams of healing light, waves of healing energy, and the powerful sound of AH are showering these people or that land.

In your mind's eye, see the beams of powerful healing light and energy waves with the AH sound enter into them, filling their bodies completely. Feel that their particular problems and the roots of those problems are completely healed. They are transformed into bodies of healing light, overflowing with boundless, blissful heat. Their minds and bodies are overflowing with the experience of peace and joy.

Again and again, send healing light and energy with the sound AH to heal them and their problems. Enjoy the images of these people absorbed in peace, joy, and well-being.

End the meditation by relaxing in open awareness of the experience, without grasping or needing to think in words about it.

11. Share the Healing Waves with the Whole Universe

In this stage of meditation, your dedication to healing others is broadened to include the entire universe. You are opening yourself up even further, as you freely send healing energy outward with no limits or restrictions.

This is the natural culmination of meditating on the "boundless" body. I can remember that when I was very young, I used to look at the sky to try and see where or whether it ended. As adults, we can all benefit from this simple sense of wonder about an endless sky and a boundless universe. In meditation, opening yourself in this way puts you in touch with a deep spirituality. It also loosens the grasping of your mind.

Purpose: Offering healing energies to the universe generates peace and joy. It broadens your perspective on life and enables you to make a real contribution to healing the world's ills. Sharing healing energies without limit magnifies the depth and scope of the healing experience.

The Guided Meditations

Again, establish in your mind the feeling of your body as radiant with amazing, colorful light, which blossoms from every one of the billions of cells in your body. Each cell is as vast as the universe. Your body, and every cell in it, is sending out beams of healing light and waves of blissful heat with the sound AH, the sound of universal love.

Visualize the whole world and think of the cries of pain, the clouds of sadness, the darkness of confusion, the flame of negative emotions, and the decay of happiness and goodness.

Now feel that bright beams of healing light and powerful healing energy waves with soothing sound are surging through every pore of your body. All this wonderful healing energy showers every being and the whole world. Every cell of every being and every particle of the whole world is filled with healing light and energy and the healing sound of AH.

Negative images and feelings, sadness and sickness, unhappy or ignorant beings, the decay of this world—all are totally healed. All negativity dissolves without a trace.

Everything is transformed into a world of light filled with healing blissful heat waves and the soothing sound of AH.

Again and again, send beams of healing light and waves of healing energy with the soothing sound of AH to heal and transform every being. Enjoy the feeling of a world totally transformed by peace and joy.

Then expand this feeling of boundless joy to the entire universe and enjoy that feeling of universal freedom, love, and peace. End the meditation with silent, open awareness of the experience.

Protect Yourself with a Healing Aura (Optional)

If you are exposed to negative forces or situations and are feeling vulnerable or sensitive, you may want to protect yourself so that you can gather your strength. In this special meditation, you can visualize a light aura in the form of an eggshell that shelters you from negativity with powerful healing energy.

Purpose: The shell of the aura protects you from real or imagined negative effects. It enforces the sense of security against self-created fears and paranoia.

Healing Meditations on the Body

To protect yourself when vulnerable, visualize in your mind's eye that waves of healing light and energy are being emitted from your body. These energies form an amazingly bright light aura, like an eggshell, around your body. Feel that nothing can penetrate this blessed energy wall, which is solid like iron and surrounded by flames of positive energy. Enjoy meditating on the image of this amazing defensive aura, with its invincible wall and protective flames.

It is also an aura of positive transmutation. Everything that touches it, including strong negativity, is transformed by its energy field into healing light and energy. Merely touching this aura causes negativity to melt like snowflakes in warm water. Enjoy the feeling of total protection and security.

Then relax into open awareness of what you are experiencing, without grasping or needing to think in words about anything.

12. *Rest in Oneness with the Healing Experience*

At the end of every meditation session, recognize what kind of healing experience you are feeling. You could be feeling peace, warmth, bliss, spaciousness, boundlessness, richness, sacredness, or strength. If you have multiple experiences, it can help to recognize the most prominent one.

The goal is to calmly enjoy the particular experience, resting in awareness of what you are feeling, without grasping at it or analyzing it or needing to think about it in words. Just remain one with the experience, in open awareness, in silence, like water that has merged in water.

Purpose: This meditation is for sowing the seed of experience of the meditation, not on the rough surface of concepts or afflicting emotions but at the deeper and calmer level of the open mind. Merging your awareness with the experience ensures the fruition of the meditation with greatest certainty. Open awareness helps unite your mind with the result of healing.

This meditation could also lead to, or be, the awareness state of the enlightened nature itself.

When you feel ready to complete your meditation, again bring your awareness to your body. Be mindful of the positive experience gener-

113

The Guided Meditations

ated by the meditation. Your body is a body of light, with billions of cells of radiant light. Each cell is as vast as the universe. Each cell is filled with healing energy with sound. As you breathe, enjoy the waves of healing energy passing through your body.

Recognize the quality of your positive experience. It could be a feeling of warmth, heat, bliss, peace, strength, spaciousness, richness, openness and light, and so on. If you have many positive experiences, recognize the most prominent one among them.

Enjoy that particular experience for a while, in total silence, by feeling it again and again.

Then think and feel that your snowflakelike mind has dissolved and merged into this oceanlike healing experience. Just be one with the particular experience, like water poured into water, and relax in it without grasping, analyzing, or needing to think in words about it.

HOW TO USE THE TWELVE STAGES IF YOU HAVE LITTLE TIME

Generally, it is important to devote the time and energy to meditate on each part of the twelve stages (which are reviewed in the accompanying box) until you can enjoy them through experience. After becoming skilled in each stage, you can meditate on the stages by selecting the parts that are important for you or by condensing all the stages. However, if you have little time and energy and wish to do only a shorter session of meditation, or if you are not yet familiar with these exercises, you can choose the parts of the stages that suit your needs. The following sets are some of those choices.

If your time and energy are limited or if you are not familiar with the healing exercises, you should meditate on just the first stage. In it, you generate peace and calmness in your body, dispel any uneasy sensations with the outgoing breath, and ground the floating mind by feeling the earth energy. Then, at the end, relax in the awareness of being one with the feeling of peace and strength, the results of the meditation.

If you feel comfortable, you can meditate on the first four stages of the exercises. Then, at the end, just relax in the awareness of being one with infinite peace and joy. The first four exercises are the basis of the twelve stages.

Healing Meditations on the Body

The Twelve Stages of Healing Meditation

Use the body as the object to be healed and as the means of healing. Heal through the four healing powers: positive images, words, feelings, and trust.

Stage 1: Bring your mind back to your body, by:
- Feeling peace in the parts of your body: head, upper body, arms and hands, lower body, legs and feet.
- Gathering any uneasy sensations into a black cloud and sensing that it leaves your body with the outgoing breath, slowly moves away, and dissolves into space.
- Connecting with the earth, grounding the floating mind.
- Uniting your body and mind in the awareness of peace.

Stage 2: Scan the anatomical details of your body to bring your mind and body closer together.

Stage 3: See your body as made of infinite individual cells to generate a sense of its expansiveness.

Stage 4: See the cells as cells of light to release stress and rigidities.

Stage 5: Enter into one cell and see the cells as vast as the universe to open boundless perception.

Stage 6: Feel that the cells are filled with healing energies in the form of heat (warmth) and bliss (joy): the source of healing.

Stage 7: Experience waves of healing light and healing energies coming from all the cells: the means of healing.

    If you have cancerous cells, then when you exhale, the energy waves from below move up; when you inhale, the energy waves from above move down; and the cancerous cells are slowly melted (burned) between the two energy waves.

Stage 8: Sing and hear the sound of the waves—AH: the force of healing.

Stage 9: Use physical movements, such as the blossoming lotus movement, to activate every part of your body as the means of creating and receiving healing energies.

Stage 10: Offer the healing waves to others.

Stage 11: Offer the healing waves to the whole universe, protecting yourself with a healing aura if you feel the need.

Stage 12: Rest in the awareness of the healing experience. Oneness.

When you have become familiar with the first four exercises, and if time permits, you should add the fifth, sixth, and seventh stages to your meditation. Then, at the end, relax in the awareness of being one with the meditative result, such as the waves of blissful heat. The fifth, sixth, and seventh exercises are the heart, the most important aspect, of the twelve stages.

If you are ready, you can add the eighth and/or ninth stage. At the end, relax in the awareness of being one with the meditative result, such as the powerful waves with sound and/or the healing movements. Although the exercises with sound and movements are the most powerful means of arousing and enhancing the healing power, you could also meditate without putting much emphasis on these exercises, as they are supplementary.

Finally, you can add the tenth and eleventh stages to your healing meditation. They are powerful means of expanding and strengthening your own healing power and sharing it with others. However, you can also meditate without these exercises, as they are auxiliary.

The twelfth stage is an important exercise for perfecting your meditation by blending yourself with it. It is done at the end of every meditation.

Further, if you are familiar with the meditations and are enjoying their results, and if your mind is calm and fully connected to your body, you could just start from the fourth stage and focus on the fifth, sixth, and seventh stages. At the end, relax in the awareness of being one with the boundless blissful heat of the body.

Of course, if you are experienced in these exercises and wish to do all the stages in a short period of time, you can do them in the following way:

1. Relax for a while. Then take a couple of deep breaths and release all tension and strain with the outgoing breath.
2. Feel the calmness in your body, from the top of your head to the soles of your feet.
3. See that your body is made of billions of cells. Feel the infinite quality of the body.
4. Then see that the cells are blossoming with light. Each cell is as vast as the universe. Each cell is overflowing with the healing energy of blissful heat. Feel that each cell is a boundless cell of healing energy.

5. Then, as you exhale and inhale, feel that every cell is sending and receiving healing energy waves. All the cells are actively sharing in the healing of the waves. Feel the wholeness and harmony of your body as the great waves of energy surge through it.
6. Then share the healing energy waves with all beings and the whole universe.
7. Finally, enjoy the feeling of whatever positive result has been produced by the meditation. Just relax in awareness of being one with the healing experience, without grasping at it or analyzing it.

SOME SPECIFIC HEALING REMEDIES

In Tibetan Buddhist meditation, healing light and warmth are the most commonly used energies. You could also choose from a variety of other approaches to healing, depending on your temperament and needs of the moment. If you have correctly diagnosed your problem, you could use the suitable means and adapt them to your needs.

The following subsections summarize various alternative healing remedies, including some that will be familiar to you and others that may be less so.

HEALING MENTAL, EMOTIONAL, AND PHYSICAL PROBLEMS

- *For a wide variety of ills of the mind and body:* Healing light, blissful heat, and blessed sound are familiar and very effective remedies.

  Visualize and feel that the problem is centered at a specific location in your body, then dispel the problem by seeing healing light, feeling blissful heat in the form of heat waves, and hearing healing sound.
- *For sad and frozen feelings:* See and feel blissful heat and believe in its healing power. First, let it purify your body; then, with your breathing, send waves of this healing energy to fill and heal your body.

  Middle and old age tend to be characterized by heightened feelings of coldness. Focus on the energy waves as healing all emotional and physical ailments related to coldness. Believe that the waves are bringing warmth, health, and strength.

117

- *For anxiety:* Think of the energy waves as endowed with the power to soothe and calm your anxieties. Feel the healing waves fill your body with calmness, strength, and joy.
- *For pain:* See and feel that your body is radiant with healing light. Think of your body as being transformed into a body of light. Believe that the pain has no opportunity to take hold or go deep, because light is translucent, insubstantial, and open. You can also use healing waves of bright light, blissful heat, and open sound.

  Or merge in oneness with the feeling of pain. Instead of grasping at how terrible the pain is, you can try to relax and simply open to it, but without judging it or labeling it as negative. This in itself can ease the pain.
- *For fear, insecurity, and weakness:* See and feel that the healing energy waves are empowering you with waves of confidence, courage, protection, strength, and warmth.
- *For anger and hatred:* Feel the soothing of energy waves endowed with love, peace, and coolness. Some people have a habitual problem with the excessive heat of anger and can benefit from meditating on healing waves that have the coolness of moonlight.
- *For attachment and craving:* See the waves as giving blessings and reaching to all with joy, generosity, and openness.
- *For confusion and darkness:* See the waves as sharp, clear light with heat, with the power to awaken clear awareness.

HEALING WITH THE COLORS OF LIGHT

In its true quality, light is manifested in five colors, which correspond to the five physical elements:

- Yellow light is the color of earth, which has the quality of solidity and generates strength.
- White light is the color of water and moisture. It harmonizes and nurtures.
- Red light is the color of fire. It is warm and magnifies power and force.
- Green light is the color of air and has the quality of lightness. It facilitates movement and development.
- Blue light is the color of space and has the quality of openness. It provides boundless space.

Healing Meditations on the Body

You could visualize a particular color of light as part of a meditation to rebuild or strengthen the energies that you most need.

HEALING PROBLEMS RELATED TO PHYSICAL STRUCTURES AND PROPERTIES

Meditation can be used to help heal physical structural problems, often in conjunction with other medical treatments:

- *For enlarged or swollen organs or channels:* See the energy waves as shrinking and reducing them to the right form and size.
- *For blockages:* See a stream of energy waves as clearing the blockages by inducing the obstructions to shrink and flushing the channels.
- *For tumors or abscesses:* See the heat of energy waves melting the tumors, which become liquid and are flushed out of your body.
- *For toxins and impurities:* See the healing waves as a stream of energy in the form of water that dilutes the toxins and impurities and purges them.
- *For fragility:* See the energy waves as invigorating and rejuvenating your body.

HEALING WITH THE ELEMENTS

In ancient Tibetan medicine, the diagnosis of a sickness and its remedy are traditionally envisioned in terms of the five elements of earth, air, fire, water, and space. The following briefly delineates this traditional approach:

- If you lack the energy of earth, see the healing waves as endowed with earth energy—heavy, firm, strong, and grounding.
- If you lack the energy of fire, see the waves as endowed with fire energy—warming, heating, and energizing.
- If you lack the energy of air, see the waves as having air energy—light, moving, and uplifting.
- If you lack the energy of water, see the waves as having the quality of water—nourishing, moistening, harmonizing, and enduring.
- If you lack the energy of space, see the waves as having the quality of space—open, spacious, and boundless, free from restrictions and conditions.

HEALING SUBSTANCES

The traditional Tibetan approach to sickness often combines prayer, meditation, and the use of external substances, including herbs and medicines. Modern medicine has given us many treatments, and we can reinforce their healing effect through meditation and positive attitude.

Healing Substances and the Healing Waves. If you are taking medicine, you can intensify its healing power by visualizing that the healing energy waves are bringing the goodness of these substances to your body. Think of the quality, potency, taste, and effect of your medicine and feel that the healing energies are intensifying the positive qualities and impact of these treatments.

Or if you are receiving radiation, meditate on the healing energies as increasing the positive effect of the treatment while repairing and healing the side effects.

Healing Substances and the Four Healing Powers. Use the four healing powers—positive seeing, recognizing, feeling, and believing—to reinforce the healing power of any positive substance, such as medicine, water, drink, food, ointment, aroma, amulets, or dressings. Think about and feel the treatment's positive effect; believe and rejoice in its healing power.

If you are interested in more information on using various objects as means of healing, you may want to refer to the predecessor of this book, *The Healing Power of Mind* (Shambhala Publications, 1996).

Healing Meditations on the Body

7

HEALING MEDITATIONS FOR SLEEPING AND WAKING

There are two crucial junctures of the day when meditation can be especially fruitful—when you are falling asleep and when you are waking up. At these times, the mind is in a transition state, and you are especially open to the power of healing. If you make a habit of experiencing peaceful feelings when the mind is naturally more open, the healing energies can take hold more deeply and firmly in your mind. Then, because you are cultivating this deeper level, it will be easier to develop a more openhearted attitude toward the rest of life. You can be more open to the experience of peace even as you are involved in your everyday activities.

Tibetan Buddhists are very interested in "in-between" states of the mind and call any such transition a *bardo*. Sleeping and waking can be considered miniature bardos. The junctures at birth and death are the major bardos, in which we enter life and leave it. Most of us feel unprepared for the transition of death and would rather not even think about it.

The qualities of the mind when you are falling asleep and waking up share some of the characteristics of death and birth. If you can directly taste and be aware of peace when falling asleep and waking, if you can practice being open during these bardos, this is an exceptional way not only to improve your life but to ready yourself for the bigger challenge of dying. So these meditations help you to be happier in life as well as gradually and gently prepare your mind for the transition that comes when you must let go of life.

You should adapt the following meditations according to your experience and needs. You may want to keep the meditations very simple and just focus on the feelings of warmth and openness in your whole body. However, if you are an experienced meditator, you could bring in more details from the healing meditations, including calling forth soothing and purifying healing energies and then experiencing a gentle version of the healing waves in rhythm with your breathing, especially your exhalations. (Note that you could also adapt the meditations from Part Three, which specifically focus on Buddhist imagery.)

MEDITATION FOR FALLING ASLEEP

During the five or ten minutes before falling asleep, use your mind's eye to see your body. See your body in its entirety, as a body of light.

Or if you wish, you could also see in more detail the parts of your body, from the top of your head to the soles of your feet. Feel that you are seeing the billions of cells of your body in the form of cells of light. Feel that every boundless cell of your body is filled with healing energy, blissful heat. Immerse yourself in the boundless healing energy of your body.

Open to the feeling of relaxation, warmth, and peace. Allow your awareness to become one with the experience, like water merging with water, without any grasping. With that feeling, go to sleep. If you wake in the middle of the night, try to immerse yourself again in the awareness of the healing energy of your boundless body and go back to sleep.

MEDITATION FOR WAKING UP

In sleep, the body and mind are harmoniously resting together, in the union of warmth and peace. As you are waking, recognize and remain

Healing Meditations on the Body

with the healing energies: simply be aware of the warmth and peace. Allow your awareness to merge for a while with these feelings.

If your mind begins jumping ahead to the day's events, obligations, or worries, gently allow these thoughts to drift away and remain instead in open awareness of peace. Take five or ten minutes to experience the union of body and mind in warmth and peace. Be at ease and relaxed in these feelings. With an open heart and mind, be at one with the moment.

If necessary, take a deep breath or two and release any tensions that you may be feeling or any impurities that you may be sensing.

Then think of your body part by part and feel the warmth and peace in each place: enjoy the natural warmth and peace of the head, the upper body, the arms and hands, the lower body, the legs and feet, and then the whole body, from the head to the soles of the feet. Simply be open; immerse yourself in a boundless feeling of healing energies. Feel warmth and openness and rest in them.

Then feel not only that your body is filled with healing energies but that there is an aura of healing energies, a tent of warmth and peace, around your body. Enjoy the healing energy atmosphere surrounding you. Bathe in that aura of warmth and peace as if you were swimming in a vast body of water like the ocean. Let your thoughts and feelings melt and merge into the ocean of healing energies, as if you have become one with it, like water merging with water. Relax in open awareness of the experience as long as you can.

Waking to the Energy of Healing Movement

To generate healing energy as you wake, you could use the physical movements described in Chapter 6, in the ninth stage of the meditations. Your mind and body are naturally in union with warmth and peace as you awaken. Simply bring your awareness to these feelings. Then practice any one, or all, of the healing movements with joyful awareness of the energy flow that very small, gradual, and subtle movements can activate. Be mindful of healing energy as you stretch and relax; expand your body with your relaxed breathing; tighten your muscles and relax; sway or rock from side to side; or very slowly move your legs in a bicycle-pedaling motion.

When you sway, you are hardly moving at all; the movement might encompass a fraction of an inch and last a minute or so. What's important in any of these movements is your open mind and heart and your total attention to feeling the energy awakening in your body as you move. Allow that feeling to expand. Rejoice in the feeling. Make an aspiration that this healing may continue all day and wish healing for all other beings, too.

OTHER MEDITATIONS TO WELCOME THE DAY

When you awake, any simple meditation of mind and body can encourage healing at a time when your awareness, like the new day, is dawning. This orientation can be an important foundation for the rest of the day.

As you are getting up to begin your morning, you can think, "I will be mindful of using this awareness of the healing energies as the basis of the day's activities." Then during the day, from time to time, recall the warmth and calmness that you felt upon awakening and let it permeate your daily activities. Let the awareness of the healing energies become the foundation of your life, like the calmness and energy of the vast ocean beneath the waves.

It is hard not to wake up with your customary worries, hopes, confusions, and ideas. However, by being mindful and aware of the healing energies as you awake, you will gradually develop a habit of waking with the right attitude.

If you can go to sleep with the awareness of peace and joy—even though you might not be aware of them in sleep itself—you could wake up with the feeling of peace and joy spontaneously. In the same way, if you could gain the experience of healing energies while you are alive, you might be able to die with that experience. Then your awareness could open to peace and joy as you are dying and even after death. Buddhists believe that such a practice during life will help immensely to secure our peaceful journey through future lives. Even if you are not Buddhist, such a practice can bring you peace of mind at the time of your death.

The following are among the many Buddhist trainings for waking:

- When you wake up, imagine that you are waking from the ignorance of sleep and now opening your mind in wisdom, the awareness of peace, joy, and light. Celebrate this feeling. You can also wish the same awakening for all beings.

Healing Meditations on the Body

- In the morning, think and feel that you have been awakened from the sleep of ignorance by the joyous voices of enlightened beings or the sounds of blessed musical instruments, such as hand drums, calling you forth to wisdom.
- Visualize and feel the arising of enlightened wisdom deities from your heart and body as you are waking up. Rejoice in the wonderful feeling that they are awakening in you the blessings of love, wisdom, and power.
- Immediately after waking, without being interrupted by other thoughts and feelings, pray and receive blessing lights or nectar from a "source of power" in the sky above you. Feel that your body and mind are purified by these blessings and that you are being transformed into a body and mind of purity, peace, and joy. Share the blessings of light or nectar with all.

DISPELLING ANXIETIES UPON SLEEPING OR WAKING

If anxieties or uneasy sensations come as you are falling asleep or waking, you can use the appropriate exercises described in Chapter 6, in the first stage of the healing meditations. For example, for floating feelings of distress, see your body as resting on the stable, solid earth. Feel your body taking on the firm, immovable qualities of the earth. Or else see yourself as a body of light—but a type of light that seems heavy, like gravity or water, making each part of your body relaxed and calm.

For anxiety or worries that make you feel tight and constricted, or for any feeling of blockages, you could see those negative energies as a dark cloud and then dispel it with light. Watch the cloud drift off harmlessly into the sky, disappearing without a trace.

Or simply merge any uneasy sensation with the warmth of the healing energies. Feel that your body is warm, calm, blissful, and peaceful. Gently guide your awareness to these feelings. If the uneasy sensations persist, merge them into the warmth and believe that they are dissolving like snow melting into water.

Or for insomnia, you could bring your awareness to your breathing. Allow your breathing to relax. Allow your thoughts and anxieties

Meditations for Sleeping and Waking

to dissolve in the natural rhythm of your breathing, especially your exhalations.

DISSOLVING ANXIETY BY MERGING IN ONENESS

At the time of waking, especially, anxieties and pains tend to be softer, since your mind is more fresh and open. So it can be easier to ease even habitual anxieties then. One way to dissolve anxieties is to merge your awareness directly with them. Merging with your feelings is considered a higher meditation than using positive feelings, and if you are relaxed and open, your mind may be receptive to this practice. If, however, you are uneasy about using this approach, go back to the more ordinary methods described earlier in this section.

Although negative feelings are painful, begin by recognizing that everything is ultimately open and peaceful in its true nature.

Instead of allowing your mind to rush after worries or push them away, simply allow the negative feelings to be. They may at that point gradually drift away. If they don't, gently ease and immerse your mind into the feeling of anxiety. Stay with the feeling instead of chasing after the complicated thoughts behind the feeling. Welcome whatever the feeling may be in a nonjudgmental way and allow the usual labels—good and bad, positive and negative—to drift away. Simply merge your awareness with whatever you are feeling.

If you open your nature and merge into unpleasant things, there is no clash of surface upon surface. The "oneness" of your awareness can ease the feeling of negativity. Rest in the feeling of oneness and openness. Then, when you feel complete, ease yourself gently and gradually into your activities, being mindful of your daily routine. As you are waking up and beginning your day, notice and rejoice in any positive feelings or any diminishing of negative feelings.

A HEALING AURA FOR
SLEEPING AND WAKING

If you are feeling emotionally vulnerable or very fearful, or if you are ill with proliferating cancer cells, you can use either of the special optional meditations described in Chapter 6 for exercises 7 and 11 (see pages 95 and 112). Both these exercises involve the visualization of

126

protective healing auras. Just before you fall asleep, it could be very helpful for you to establish a connection with whichever meditation fits your situation.

You may wish to do the meditation fully at this time, in a way that is comfortable and relaxed. Or you can simply remember and reestablish in your mind and body the positive feelings of the healing meditation that you did earlier in the day. Feel the warmth and healing energy again in your body and feel that the healing aura has formed and is again firmly in place.

Think that these healing energies are protecting and healing you as you fall asleep. Believe and be glad that the healing will continue all night long.

Then, when you wake up, immediately remember that the healing aura has been with you while you slept. Be glad for the peace and healing power that have been working all night long. Feel that the healing is continuing even now as your awareness dawns upon waking. In this way, the cycle of healing is reinforced night and day.

Part Three

Buddhist meditations to heal mind and body

8

MEDITATION ON THE HEALING BUDDHA

INTRODUCTION

Until now, I have emphasized the universality of the approach to healing mind and body. Anyone can practice the meditations in Part Two, without believing in Buddhism, even if he or she has another religious belief or none at all.

It's not necessary to use Buddhist images for meditation to be effective. However, if you are a practicing Buddhist or are interested in Buddhism, then it makes sense to use the wealth of devotional images from a tradition that has been developed and refined over many centuries. If you do, you will be walking along a path well trodden by many enlightened sages.

The underlying principles for the meditations in Part Three are the same as I've already discussed. You are healing problems through the power of your own mind. That power can transform negative mental images, thoughts, feelings, and habitual patterns into the positive qualities of a peaceful mind.

The focal point is traditional Tibetan Buddhist imagery. You will be invoking the healing blessings of enlightened buddha nature, which is your birthright and that of others. Again, your main allies in calling upon the transforming power of your mind are the four healing powers: seeing, thinking, feeling, and believing. You will see the blessed images in your mind, recognize their power through sacred words or prayers, feel their positive spiritual qualities, and trust in their blessings with confidence.

Buddhist meditation is rich in variety. There are so many approaches and techniques from which to choose. Here, you will be focusing on the body as the object to be healed—and also as the means to bring healing to the mind. These meditations can help you enjoy a happier life and could also lead to higher realization.

With pure perception, you see the source of healing blessings as the enlightened buddha presence. With devotion, you believe in the power of mind to transform your ordinary body into the form of an enlightened body and an enlightened abode.

DEVOTIONAL MEDITATION

Devotional meditation is a means of awakening and expressing our own inner resources, which are essential for healing.

To heal our minds and bodies, we visualize images of the Buddha. We think of and feel the presence of these Healing Buddhas, the enlightened ones to whom we pray, and believe in their healing power. We invoke and enjoy their blessings.

This may sound like idol worship, but it really is not. In Buddhism, external sources and mental objects are a means to an end. The ultimate source of healing is our minds, not the external objects, which of themselves have no power to save us or change our fate. The Buddha said:

> *I have shown you*
> *The way that leads beyond the pain of craving.*
> *[But] Buddha is [just] a guide.*
> *You are the one who must take the steps.*[1]

Accepting blessed objects as the means of training is what Buddhists call "skillful means." Blessed objects inspire and support us, but

Buddhist Meditations

the main factor is not the objects. It is the way we see, think, and feel about these objects, the strength of our trust in them, that helps us advance along the positive path of healing.

The whole universe—mind and body, the earth and stars, time and space—is all one in having the ultimate peace of enlightened nature. Water in the ocean, in a bottle, and in a cup appears in different forms but is one in being water. Enlightened nature is the nature of you, me, and the whole universe, though we appear different. Enlightened nature is beyond the limits of images, words, or concepts as they are contrived and designated by the dualistic mind, which thinks of things as "subject" and "object" rather than omnisciently realizing their unified nature.

If the whole universe is one in enlightened nature, ultimate peace and joy, and if it is the true nature of all of us, then why do we need to practice devotion for healing?

By grasping at "self," our ordinary minds limit our perspective to "I" and "you," "this" and "that." This grasping quality of mind confines us to a prisonlike cycle of confusion, limitation, and pain.

Meditation loosens this grasping and breaks down the mental and emotional barriers between "I" and "you," "me" and "others." It releases doubts and fears. The power of devotion brings a blessing shower that can heal emotional and mental ills and encourage the blossoming of enlightened mind in us.

So as long as we are emotional and dualistic, we must welcome the external sources of blessed objects as a support for healing. If our minds are not trained and developed, we are like a toddler learning to walk. We must take baby steps and hold onto mother's hand to stand up until our muscles are strong enough that we can walk on our own.

Devotion is a mind full of blossoming energy rooted in trust, in which there are no doubts. It is trust in the Healing Buddhas as the ultimate source of healing. It is trust in meditation as the perfect path of healing and in those who are on the healing path as the true supports for our journey.

If we have trust and faith in these positive objects, every step that we take will lead us in the right direction, and we can be fully confident that our final goals will be reached. Guru Padmasambhava, the founder of Buddhism in Tibet, said:

> *If your mind is free from doubts, wishes will be achieved.*
> *If you have total trusting faith, blessings will come to you.*[2]

Without the rays of the sun, the snow upon the mountains can't melt into streams of water. Without devotion to the Healing Buddhas from the depth of our hearts, no healing blessings can come into our lives. Devotion loosens our grasping and allows our true nature to shine forth and blossom. Kyobpa Rinpoche, founder of the Drigungpa Kagyudpa school, emphasizes the importance of devotion:

> *From the snow-mountain–like master . . . ,*
> *Without the touch of the rays of sunlike devotion,*
> *The streamlike blessing will not flow.*
> *So exert your mind in the training of devotion.*[3]

If we do not have devotional trust, even if the Healing Buddha in person were standing in front of us, we would receive hardly any benefit. For our minds, which are the only key to our spiritual blossoming, would not open to the opportunity. This is why a Tibetan proverb says:

> *From whomever one sees as a Buddha*
> *Blessings are received as from a Buddha.*
> *From whomever one sees as a fool*
> *Effects come as from a fool.*

The enlightened nature, ultimate peace and joy, is omnipresent; it is in all of us. Training in devotion is a powerful way to uncover that nature. Seeing the image of a Buddha as endowed with blessed qualities can transform our minds. If we can see and feel the enlightened qualities of this object, we will open our minds to healing. If we can think of the object as blessed and trust in its power, a peaceful and joyful feeling will spontaneously blossom in our minds.

If we can't open to external objects as a source of healing, it will be hard to appreciate our own positive inner qualities. Relying on blessed objects is a way to eliminate habits of negative perception and emotion. Then we will have a chance to regain our confidence and awaken to the experience of peace and joy.

Certain Buddhist trainings use the act of bowing down or prostrating to a blessed object or being as an expression of devotion. This is a simple but powerful way of surrendering the ego, for it is our grasping at ego that keeps us from ever opening up to positive perceptions. In

Buddhist Meditations

the guided meditations we shall do, we don't physically bow, but the intention is the same. We are letting go of our grasping minds and opening to healing.

THE POWER OF THE HEALING BUDDHAS

Everyone and everything is a manifestation of buddha nature. That is the highest understanding of buddhahood in its true nature. But as a first step, we need to identify a blessed object to help us experience the positive qualities of mind. As a skillful means in helping our meditation, we need the image and presence of a Buddha on whom to rely.

There are numerous names and personifications of Buddhas endowed with various significances—for example, Pranjaparamita for wisdom, Tara for protection from fears, Manjushri for scholarship, Avalokiteshvara for compassion, Vajrapani for power, Vajrasattva for purification, Sarasvati for speech, Vasudhara for prosperity, Guru Padmasambhava for spiritual accomplishments, Yeshey Tsogyal for great bliss, and our spiritual teachers for blessings. We can use the form and name of a Buddha that suits our needs or that inspires our minds.

In this book, we are using the image of the Healing Buddha as the source of blessing. His name in Sanskrit is Bhaishajya-guru baidūrya-prabha-raja. It means the Lord of Lapis Light, the Master of Healing. *Lapis* comes from lapis lazuli, a bright blue stone that is radiant with light.

According to Buddhist scriptures, the special quality of the Healing Buddha is the power inspired through his twelve aspirations or vows,[4] which arc as follows:

1. May all beings attain the physical endowments of a supreme being by the touch of the lapis light of my body.
2. May all beings who are in darkness enjoy light and live with virtues by the touch of my lapis light.
3. May infinite beings enjoy great leisure through the inexhaustible wealth created by the power of my skillful means and wisdom.
4. May I be able to lead all beings along the path of enlightenment.
5. By hearing my name, may all beings live in pure moral conduct and may none stray into inferior realms.
6. By hearing my name, may all beings recover from their physical disabilities and enjoy good health forever.

135

7. By hearing my name, may all who are destitute obtain protection and care and live in prosperity.

8. By hearing my name, may all women who are suffering and wishing for liberation be liberated.

9. May I be able to release all beings from Mara's traps and lead them to the enjoyment of pure view.

10. By the power of my merits, may all be free from the tyranny of rulers.

11. May I be able to nourish all who are hungry and thirsty with the gifts of food, drink, and the nectar of dharma.

12. May I be able to adorn all who are naked and cold with rich garments and ornaments and serve them with great entertainments.[5]

In these meditations, it is important to know that we are not invoking the Healing Buddha as an individual enlightened one but as the embodiment of all the enlightened ones: all Buddhas, divinities, saints, and sages. We are seeing him as the manifestation of our own true nature and qualities and the true nature and qualities of the whole universe.

VISUALIZING AND PRAYING TO THE HEALING BUDDHA

As background to this meditation, it is useful to know some details about the image of the Healing Buddha and its significance.

Each aspect of the Healing Buddha's image—the form, posture, color, and gesture—has its own special meaning and its particular spiritual significance and quality. Seeing and understanding these spiritual qualities encourages them to arise in us. We develop the habit of seeing the rich and full spiritual quality of everything around us, and in doing so, we are sowing the seeds that can awaken the enlightened qualities of the mind.

Detailed visualization of the image helps us to generate a focused state of mind. It helps overly intellectual people to use their gift of active mind positively. And it helps overly dull people to sharpen and awaken their minds.

During the meditation, we try to visualize the image of the Buddha as clearly as we find comfortable. But we don't worry if we lack experience and skill in visualization. What really matters is the feelings that the prayers and images evoke in us and our trust in the power of the meditation. We use the feelings to call up in our minds an image of the Healing Buddha that is simple but heartfelt. If we feel the warmth and presence of the Healing Buddha, that in itself is very healing.

Remember, too, that artistic renderings such as those in this book are meant as an aid. A picture or statue may inspire us, teach us, or help as a starting point for visualization, but we shouldn't feel limited by it. What matters in visualization is the thought of being in the presence of the Healing Buddha and the warmth, peace, and joy that we feel in our hearts.

At the beginning of the meditation, we will be visualizing a totally open clear blue sky out of which appears the seat of the Healing Buddha, a huge blossoming lotus (see the accompanying illustration). On it is a shining, clear moon disc. Then the Healing Buddha appears from the open sky. This visualization symbolizes the total openness of the Healing Buddha, his immaculate purity, and omnipresent compassion. Such images help us to experience openness and purity as the foundation of the meditation and to see and feel that buddha nature is everywhere and in everything.

On the moon disc sits the Healing Buddha in contemplative posture. His body is adorned with 112 excellent physical signs to symbolize the perfection of his merits and wisdom. The richness and perfection of the imagery remind us of our own perfect inner nature and help to awaken our inner Healing Buddha.

Our main focus of prayer is the Healing Buddha, the Lord of Lapis Light, but we are also praying to the infinite Buddhas, bodhisattvas, and sages in male and female form whom we also see as sources of healing. So when we say "the Healing Buddha," we are referring to the Lord of Lapis Light, and when we say "the Healing Buddhas," we are referring to all the enlightened ones, the sources of healing to whom we are praying.

We are using an infinite number of images of Buddhas, or enlightened ones, because many of us get more inspiration if there are numerous divine presences before us. However, if we prefer, we may have only one Healing Buddha as the source of healing blessings. The Healing Buddha is an image and a name of one Buddha, but in his true quality, he embodies all the enlightened ones.

By seeing, thinking, feeling, and believing in the presence of the Healing Buddhas before us, devotional energies arise in us and melt all

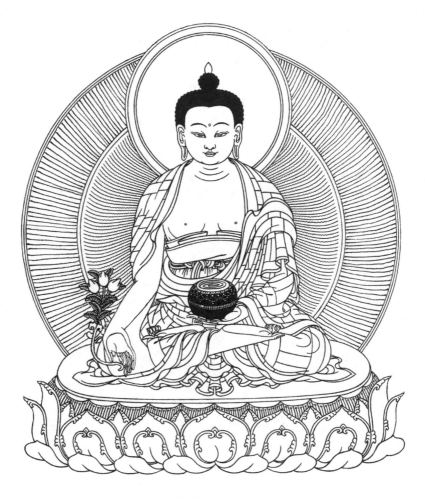

our worries and pain. Our prayer is to let the qualities of healing, peace, and joy shine in us through the force of healing energy, blissful heat. We pray for the birth of the union of openness and wisdom in our minds.

As we pray to the Healing Buddha and all the enlightened ones surrounding him, we will sing or chant the name-prayer (or in Sanskrit, *dharani*) aloud or in our minds, loudly or quietly. We will repeat the name-prayer many times in a sweet voice with a reverent heart.

Prayers are the means of invoking the compassionate minds of the Healing Buddhas and channeling physical and mental energies into healing energies. The sound of the name-prayer helps to transmute all our problems into the awareness of oneness, the union of peace and joy.

Prayers are exercises that enable our minds to open themselves in earnest devotion to the power of the Healing Buddha. Prayers open the doors of our hearts and minds for the blessings of the Healing Buddha to enter. Prayers are celebrations of our mental and physical joy at being in the presence of the Healing Buddha. Prayers are the affirmation of our total trust and confidence in the Healing Buddha. Prayers are the channel by which we unify ourselves with the Healing Buddha.

For this meditation, I am going to present the complete name-prayer of the Healing Buddha. But we could also say any prayer—any positive words, phrase, or syllable such as AH—instead of the name-prayer, if that is more inspiring for invoking healing devotion and healing energies. Chanting the name-prayer is more effective, but if reciting it produces uneasiness, we could simply chant "AIIIIIII AIIIIIII AHHHH" as the prayer to the Healing Buddha and to all enlightened ones. The sound AII is the essence of transcendental wisdom, the very sound and mother of all the enlightened ones.

Here is the name-prayer, or dharani, of the Healing Buddha,[6] along with its translation:

Tibetanized Sanskrit:
Tad-ya-tha om bhe-kha-dzye bhe-kha-dzye ma-ha-bhe-kha-dzye ra-dza sa-mud-ga-te so-ha.

Sanskrit:
Tadyatha om bhaishajye bhaishajye mahabhaishajye raja samud-gate svaha.

Meditations on the Healing Buddha

The following are several possible free/interpretive translations of the name-prayer:

Thus, hail to the body, speech, and mind of the Buddhas: the King of Healing, of Healing, of Great Healing, the Fully Exalted One.

Thus, O King of Healing, of Healing, of Great Healing, the Fully Exalted One—may your blessings consecrate us.

Thus, hail to the body, speech, and mind of the Buddhas: King in [the field of] Healing, in Healing, in Great Healing, the Fully Exalted One—may your blessings consecrate us.

The scriptures contain various versions of the name-prayer of the Healing Buddha, which differ in wording and length, but the form presented here is common in many Tibetan Buddhist texts. The meaning of this name-prayer can be interpreted in different ways and at different levels. As always, what is most important is the feeling of warmth and trust evoked through the prayer.

RECEIVING BLESSINGS FROM THE HEALING BUDDHAS

By positive seeing, thinking, feeling, and believing, you will receive the healing blessing light and energy from the sources of healing, the Healing Buddhas.

Develop trust that the compassionate Healing Buddhas are present before you and that they have the power to grant healing. Believe that they are sending their wisdom, compassion, and power in the form of healing light, energies, and sound and that these blessings have the power to heal all your ills. Feel and believe that these blessing lights are endowed with powerful, blissful heat, the energy that heals your ills.

In this meditation, you will be employing blessing light and energy, blissful heat, and the sound of the Healing Buddha's name-prayer as the means of healing. But you could also use water, fire, air, earth, space, smell, taste, and/or touch with healing energy and sound as the means of healing, depending on your needs.

Or instead of light, you can use nectar as the means of healing.

Visualize and feel that a stream of nectar is flowing to you from the Healing Buddha's nectar bowl and/or from all the Healing Buddhas.

In this meditation, use the power of your imagination and senses to increase the effect of the healing. See and feel that the stream of nectar has a powerful and sweet medicinal taste and aroma. The unconditional love of the Healing Buddhas is coming to you in the form of a stream of medicinal nectar. It is warm and blissful. It has the buddha power of totally healing all your mental and physical ills at their roots.

You will visualize that the nectar enters the top of your head. The force of the nectar flood slowly washes down all the filth and purges it through the lower doors and the pores of your body. Your body is totally cleansed of the filth and purified, like a bottle washed clean. First, it washes away all your mental, emotional, and physical toxins and suffering in the form of filth. Then, more nectar enters and fills your whole body and mind, transforming you with the blessing of the nectar and heat and bliss.

HEALING YOUR ILLS BY MEDITATING ON THE HEALING BUDDHAS

If you are feeling icelike coldness and stonelike hardness in your body and mind, meditating on a warm, streamlike flow of blessing light and blissful heat can help you dissolve and melt your problems.

Feel the experience of heat and bliss accompanied by feelings of invincible power and strength that overcome every problem like the force of sunlight banishing all darkness from the earth by the mere touch of its rays. Use the power of trust to release mental and emotional pressures, stress, and worries. During the time of the meditation, totally believe that these problems are banished forever as you merge with oceanlike peace and joy.

Allow all the rigid concepts and feelings to merge into the ocean of blessing energy, blissful heat, like snowflakes into water, leaving no separation or boundaries between good and bad, this and that, I and you.

In this meditation, you are visualizing your mental and physical problems in the form of darkness. But you could also visualize your problems as tumors, flames, ice, or filth or as they are in their actual form in the place where you feel them.

Then you could visualize the healing blessings in the form that would be appropriate for healing these ills. If you visualize your problem as a tumor, for example, the healing blessings could take the form of laserlike light to cut the tumor to pieces and flush it out.

Also, a healer could receive healing blessings from the Healing Buddha and channel them to another person through his or her hands.

Although you may feel the healing energies physically, it is actually your mind that is generating the energies. So your mind is being healed as well as your body. If your mind is filled with healing energies, all your perceptions can become one with the healing. This carries over to the rest of your life, allowing you to become happier and more peaceful.

MERGING IN ONENESS

Merging in oneness allows the benefits of the healing meditation to deepen in our minds and bodies. After the stages of visualization are complete, we simply open to the most prominent positive feeling we are having, enjoying the experience for a while without thinking of anything else.

Finally, we just remain in a state of awareness, without grasping at a conceptual view of our meditation or anything else. As we open, our awareness merges with experience, so that the three aspects of the ordinary mind—the subject, or mind; the object, such as joy; and the action, feeling joy—become one. We simply remain in awareness of the feeling of joy, in oneness, like water in water.

For some meditators, open awareness merges all concepts and feelings into the single infinite healing blessing, the union of heat, bliss, peace, and joy. Then there are no conceptual and emotional distinctions, limitations, or afflictions to create pain and excitement, good and bad. In the state of ultimate healing, all are one in ultimate peace and joy.

Generally, the meditation on oneness is considered the most profound and the summit of all Buddhist meditations. In their true nature and quality, our minds and bodies are the union of peace and power, wisdom and light. This union is the presence of universal buddhahood.

When we realize the true nature, buddha wisdom, all phenomena around us will be awakened as the power or light of wisdom, which is the Buddha pure land. We won't need to purify them, for they are pure. Then all our activities will become divine manifestations for the benefit of all.

Meditators with deep experience in this higher meditation don't necessarily need to practice the healing visualizations. For most of us, however, the purpose of meditating on oneness is mainly to bring the positive impact of healing visualizations to a deeper and calmer level of the mind, where there is less mental conflict and emotional turmoil. So ending the session with such a meditation increases the certainty of achieving effective results with maximum benefits.

MAINTAINING THE RIGHT ATTITUDE IN MEDITATING

As you are getting ready to begin, think to yourself, "I am going to pray and meditate on the Healing Buddha to heal the sufferings and confusion of all beings." According to Buddhism, if you start meditation with the attitude of doing it for the happiness and enlightenment of an infinite number of beings, the power of your meditation is multiplied. Its effect will be greatly increased, and it will benefit not only you but many others as well.

THE TWELVE STAGES OF MEDITATION ON THE HEALING BUDDHA

1. Bring Your Mind Back to Your Body

The stage of meditation in which you bring your mind back to your body is the same as described in Chapter 6. It's presented here again, in a somewhat abbreviated form, to allow you to see it alongside the other stages of meditation that focus specifically on Buddhist imagery.

Bringing Calmness to the Body. Feelings such as calmness and peace are concepts created by the mind and experiences felt by the mind. So let your mind generate the thought and feeling of calmness in your body.

Think and feel that your body is very calm. Your whole body is filled with calmness.

Now slowly go through your body, devoting a few minutes to each part, starting from the soles of your feet.

Feel calmness in the soles of your feet. Feel calmness in your feet.

143

Feel calmness in your legs. Feel calmness in your abdomen. Feel calmness in your chest. Feel calmness in your shoulders. Feel calmness in your arms. Feel calmness in your hands. Feel calmness in your neck. Feel calmness in your head. Feel calmness in your brain.

Feel that your whole body is filled with calmness. Your whole body is one in total calmness and peace. Feel not only that your body is filled with calmness but that it has become the body of calmness.

Think and feel that all those around you are filled with calmness. The whole room where you are sitting is filled with calmness. The whole village, city, or town is filled with calmness. Finally, the whole universe is filled with calmness. There is nothing but calmness wherever your mind goes. The universe is a universe of calm and peace. Enjoy the feeling of boundless calm, the universal calmness.

Dispelling Gross or Subtle Uneasy Sensations. At this point, if you are experiencing any uneasy sensation—such as boredom, suffocation, anxiety, or pain—then, with a calm disposition, acknowledge and recognize the presence of that uneasy sensation.

Now find where that uneasy sensation is located or where you feel it is mainly centered in your body. Briefly think and feel that any uneasy sensation that you might be experiencing in other parts of your body is gathered at the place where it is centered.

Then take a couple of deep and forceful breaths. Think and feel that the uneasy sensation is expelled with your outgoing breath: "Haaa! . . . Haaa!! . . . Haaa!!!" The uneasy sensation is completely expelled from your body, leaving no trace behind.

Finally, think and feel that the uneasy sensation is totally gone. Feel the freedom from that sensation in your body. Let your body feel relaxed and calm. Enjoy the calmness and peace, the absence of that sensation. Your whole body is relaxed, refreshed, and awakened in peace and calmness.

Grounding the Floating Mind. To deal with floating sensations, focus your awareness on the touch of your body on your seat or the floor. Feel the touch of your body on the seat or floor.

Now think that you are not just sitting on the seat or floor but that you are sitting on and touching the earth. Feel the touch of your body on the earth.

Think that you are touching the earth energies, such as firmness, solidity, heaviness, and unmovable, unshakable strength. Feel your body touching these energies. Feel the firmness, solidity, and heaviness of the earth.

Feel that your body is being filled with the earth energies: firmness, solidity, heaviness, and unmovable strength. Your whole body is filled completely with earth energy.

Feel that the peace and calmness of your body and the firmness and heaviness of the earth are united in your body. Your body is filled with calmness and firmness. Your body is a body of calmness and firmness.

Your mind is one with your body, and your mind and body are in harmony with calmness and firmness.

Being at One with the Feeling of Calm. When you feel complete in the exercise of bringing mind back to body, notice and recognize the feeling of boundless calm that has come to your body. Enjoy the feeling of peace and joy generated by this calmness and firmness.

Then relax in the state of open awareness of the feeling of peace and joy, joyful peace, without grasping at it or needing to think in words about it. Remain in oneness with joyful peace, in total silence, like water in water, as long as you can.

Note: At this point, you might want to scan the anatomical details of the body, as described in Chapter 6, exercise 2.

2.   *Visualize the Healing Buddhas with Devotion*

Imagine that you are sitting at some lofty spot such as a mountaintop, looking at the vast, clear, boundless blue sky. With your mind's eye, see the clarity, openness, and boundlessness of the sky or of whatever mental object you are seeing. Enjoy the feeling of vast and totally open nature for a while.

Now, in the middle of that open sky, see a huge blossoming lotus arising spontaneously. It is a beautiful lotus with thousands of colorful petals blossoming boundlessly. It is fresh with dew and is sending out sweet fragrance in all directions. Do not just see but feel in yourself the blossoming quality of the lotus that you're seeing. Feel in yourself the enchanting beauty of the lotus. Feel its freshness and purity.

At the center of this brilliant lotus, visualize a clear, shining moon disc. It is not round like a ball but flat like a cushion. It is clear and shining, emitting rays of cool light. Feel in yourself the shining quality of the moon that you are seeing. Feel the clarity and the purity of the

145

moon. Feel its coolness, which eases the burning heat of your mind and body.

Recognize that the lotus and moon, arising out of openness, are symbols of the open nature of the Healing Buddha.

Now see the Healing Buddha himself appearing from the open sky to take his place on the moon seat. The Healing Buddha arises in immaculate openness, blossoming joy, and everlasting peace.

The Healing Buddha is a radiant youth with a body of rainbowlike blue light. See the healing Buddha in an aura of colorful and beautiful light, adorned with the physical attributes of a supreme being. His presence is powerful like a mountain of lapis lazuli or sapphire, and he shines as if touched by the rays of thousands of suns.

The Healing Buddha is dressed in three simple ascetic robes (the lower garment, upper shawl, and outer shawl) made of colorful light. His luminous body radiates blessing light in all directions, dispelling the darkness of confusion, sadness, and pain and showering the universe with the light of joy and peace.

He sits majestically and firmly in meditative posture, like a mountain, symbolizing the unchanging equanimity of buddha nature.

With his right hand resting on his right knee in a supreme gesture of giving, he holds a myrobalam (arura), the king of medicinal herbs, by the stem, between his thumb and index finger. This gesture symbolizes his power and his vow to bestow supreme attainments on others and to heal all sicknesses and their causes through the power of his healing wisdom, as medicinal fruits and plants cure diseases.

With his left hand resting on his lap in a contemplative gesture, he holds an ascetic's bowl filled with healing ambrosia. This gesture symbolizes his unwavering attainment of the supreme wisdom, the ultimate peace and joy, through the power of ultimate healing, as nectar is compounded of all medicines.

The Healing Buddha is looking with a contemplative glance at each of us, all the time, unblinking, with his loving doe eyes. This symbolizes his omniscient wisdom and omnipresent compassion.

He is youthful like a sixteen-year-old, for he is at the peak of youth, untempered by decay and change.

His face is filled with a beautiful smile of joy, as his enlightened mind is forever beyond any pain and confusion.

The whole space in front of you is filled with colorful rainbow lights. The Healing Buddha sits in the midst of this radiant, blossoming light, encircled by an ocean of male and female Buddhas, bodhisatt-vas, and divine beings, like the moon in the midst of numerous stars and planets in a clear, dark night sky.

Think and believe that every Buddha, bodhisattva, and divine being present before you is a Healing Buddha, as they are enlightened and have the power to heal all sufferings.

Think and believe that the Healing Buddhas are omnisciently wise and know everything that happens—in your life and in every realm of the world—simultaneously and without confusion. Feel that you are seeing the Buddhas in their omniscient wisdom.

Their infinite compassion is open to the whole universe and reaches every single being, as a mother reaches out to her only child with un-conditional love. Feel the touch of the love of the Buddhas.

Their boundless power heals the problems of all beings and fulfills the needs and wishes of anyone whose mind is opened by devotion.

The Healing Buddhas are not some beings outside yourself but are the reflection, the manifestation, of your own true nature. The true nature and pure qualities of your own mind—the ultimate peace, total joy, and omniscient wisdom—have arisen as the Healing Buddhas be-fore your open mind.

The Healing Buddhas are not separate from the true nature of the world. The world is one with the omniscience, wisdom, and omnipres-ence of the Buddhas. The Healing Buddhas are the pure, positive im-ages, sounds, and feelings arisen from and reflected by the true nature and quality of buddhahood, the true nature and qualities of the uni-verse. Feel the oneness of the Healing Buddhas and the universe.

Finally, enjoy the feeling of being in the presence of the loving, powerful Healing Buddhas. Enjoy the feeling of peace and joy gener-ated by being in the presence of the Healing Buddhas.

Then relax in open awareness of peace and joy, joyful peace, in total silence, without grasping at your feelings or analyzing or needing to think in words.

3. With Prayers, Invoke the Blessings of the Healing Buddhas

Develop a strong devotion to the Healing Buddhas from the depth of your heart, thinking and believing that these Buddhas present before you are not just forms created by your mind but are the actual presence of the Healing Buddhas.

147

Feel that devotional energies, the energies of heat and bliss, are bursting from your heart, from your mind, and from your body. Devotional energies are causing you to open and blossom into wholeness, in celebration, in boundless celebration.

Feel and believe that your mind and body are open and have become vessels to receive the blessing energies from the Buddhas.

Visualize and think that the whole earth is filled with all kinds of beings—human beings, animals, birds, insects, visible and invisible beings. They are all—with cheerful faces, joyful wide-open eyes, and reverent hearts—looking with totally focused, one-pointed minds at the compassionate and powerful face of the Buddha and the Healing Buddhas surrounding him.

Think and feel that they are all joining you in singing the name-prayer of the Healing Buddha with a soothing sound of celebration. The whole universe is filled with one sound, the sound of this pure name-prayer, in thunderous sweet, soothing melodies. Hear all the sounds of the world—such as the sound of people, traffic, birds, and wind—as the sounds of devotional energies.

Feel that the energies of the devotional prayers are opening the minds of every being in total devotional joy, as sunlight causes all the flowers to blossom.

Feel and believe that the energy of your devotion and prayer, your heartfelt calling, is invoking the compassionate minds of the Healing Buddhas.

With total trust, and feeling the energy of devotion, sing the name-prayer or the AH syllable as the prayer, from the depth of your heart in sweetest melodies, filling the whole universe.

You could chant or sing the name-prayer (dharani) of the Healing Buddha in either Tibetanized Sanskrit or pure Sanskrit:

Tibetanized Sanskrit:
Tad-ya-tha om bhe-kha-dzye bhe-kha-dzye ma-ha-bhe-kha-dzye ra-dza sa-mud-ga-te so-ha.

Sanskrit:
Tadyatha om bhaishajye bhaishajye mahabhaishajye raja samud-gate svaha.

The following are free/interpretive translations of the name-prayer:

Buddhist Meditations

Thus, O King of Healing, of Healing, of Great Healing, the Fully Exalted One—may your blessings consecrate us.

Thus, hail to the body, speech, and mind of the Buddhas: the King of Healing, of Healing, of Great Healing, the Fully Exalted One.

If you prefer to sing the AH syllable, then sing this blessed sound with heartfelt devotion as you exhale, as follows: "AHHHHHHHHHHHH AHHHHHHHHHHHHHH AHHHHHHHHHHHHH."

Finally, enjoy the boundless power of the energy of devotion and prayer. Enjoy the peace and joy created as a result.

Then relax in the state of open peace and joy, the joyful peace, in total silence, without grasping at it or thinking about it.

4.   *Receive the Healing Blessings*

See and feel the presence of the Healing Buddha in the midst of infinite Healing Buddhas, all thinking of you and looking at you with love, wisdom, and power.

Think and feel that your mind and body are blossoming and opening with the energy of devotion and devotional prayer, blissful heat. Devotional energy has made you an open vessel to receive the blessings of the Healing Buddhas.

Simultaneously, think and believe that the prayers have invoked the compassionate and powerful wisdom minds of the Healing Buddhas and that as a result, they are sending you blessings.

Visualize that beams of blessing light of various colors are emitted from different parts of the body of the Healing Buddha and the infinite Healing Buddhas and are shining upon you.

These beams of light are like a stream of nectar.[7] They are the beams of love, wisdom, and power that the Healing Buddhas are sending to you as their blessings.

These beams of light are not just beautiful, pure forms of light; they are the light of heat and bliss, powerful, blissful heat. These beams of light are not inanimate. They are the wisdom minds of the Buddhas in the form of blessing light.

Think and feel that the shower of blessing light is touching the skin of your body, front and back, and from the top of your head to the soles of your feet. Feel the blessing energies, heat and bliss, the blissful heat of the blessing light.

149

Now, with your mind's eye, look inside your body. Your body is totally dark inside. See and feel that this darkness is your problems. This darkness is your mentality of tightness, rigidity, and grasping. It is the afflicting emotions of confusion, greed, and hatred. It is the feeling of sadness, anxiety, insecurity, and pain. It is the sickness and disease of your body. It is the impurities of your energy. See and feel that this darkness of your body is the problems that you want to heal. Briefly feel the sensation of your problems in this darkness.

Then think and feel that the beams of bright light are entering your body through every pore. Your body is filled with the flow of blessing light. Your whole body, from the top of your head to the soles of your feet, is filled with the blessing light.

See the amazing brightness of the blessing light that has totally filled your body. As your body is filled with the blessing light, feel also that your body is filled with powerful heat and bliss, blissful heat. Feel that blessing energies have filled every cell of your body. They have filled every corner of every cell.

Think and believe that the blessing powers of the Healing Buddhas, in the form of bright light and powerful energy, have entirely filled your body. All the darkness of your life is dispelled from your body, totally, without leaving even a trace, as if thousands of suns had arisen in your body. All your problems, in the form of darkness, have vanished completely.

(You could add, if you wish, that the blessing light and blissful heat are melting the icelike coldness and hardness of your rigid mind into a soft, peaceful, and warm feeling. The blessing energies melt all coldness into a flowing, healing, warm stream that washes away all the frigidities of pain and sadness.)

Finally, enjoy the feeling of peace and joy, joyful peace, and freedom from all imperfections.

Then relax in open awareness of the peace and joy, joyful peace, in total silence, without grasping at it or thinking about it.

Here's an alternative meditation that calls forth healing nectar as the blessing:

First, with your mind's eye, look inside your body. Your body is filled with filth. Think of whatever problems you have—the pain or distress of your mind or diseases of your body, such as tumors, injuries, clogging of blood vessels, dead cells, impure blood or energies. Visualize and feel those particular problems in the form of filth where you believe they are located or else visualize and feel them as accurately as possible in their actual form and location.

Think and feel that the filth that you are seeing in your body is the manifestation of the problems, with their various causes and effects. Think that this filth is the tight, rigid, and grasping habits that condition your mind. It is the confusion, greed, and hatred that afflict your emotions. It is the feelings of sadness, anxiety, insecurity, and pain that torment your mind. It is the sicknesses and diseases that ruin your body. It is the impurities of your blood and energy that defile your circulatory system and make it fail. Briefly feel the sensation of your problems in this filth.

Now, in the space before you, visualize and feel the presence of the Healing Buddha in the midst of infinite Healing Buddhas looking at you with love, wisdom, and power.

Think and feel that your mind and body are blossoming and opening with the energies of prayers and devotion, blissful heat. Devotional energies have made you an open vessel to receive the blessings of the Healing Buddhas.

Think and believe that your prayers have invoked the compassionate and powerful wisdom minds of the Healing Buddhas.

Visualize and feel that as the result of your devotion, a stream of healing nectar comes from the body of the Healing Buddha. It also streams from the myrobalam (arura) in his right hand, which is the king of medicinal herbs, and from the ascetic's bowl filled with healing ambrosia in his left hand.

The stream of nectar is the love, wisdom, and power of the Healing Buddha appearing in the form of healing nectar that has the power to heal all your problems by its mere touch.

It is a stream of nectar that radiates light and is filled with powerful heat and bliss.

The stream of nectar is not inanimate. It is the wisdom mind of the Healing Buddhas appearing in the form of nectar.

Then visualize and feel that the stream of blessing nectar radiating light enters your body through the crown of your head. Your body is filled with the flow of warm blessing nectar like a pot being filled with water. Your whole body, from the top of your head to the soles of your feet, is filled with amazingly bright and clear blessing nectar. Every cell of your body is filled with the powerful heat and bliss of the blessing nectar. Every corner of every cell is completely filled with nectar.

Visualize and feel that all the filth that you have in your body is slowly being melted by the bright, warm, and blissful blessing nectar, like ice in warm water. The stream of nectar with melted filth floods down and exits through the lower doors of your body. The filth of your body is melted totally, leaving no trace behind. Then the healing nectar with the purified fluid travels to the earth and dissolves and evaporates into empty, vast outer space. See and feel that all your problems have totally vanished.

Now think and feel that your pure body is being filled up again with the medicinal nectar flooding from the Healing Buddhas. Your body, and every one of its cells, is filled to capacity with the medicinal nectar. Your body has become a body totally filled with medicinal nectar of the Healing Buddhas with amazing healing energies, heat, and bliss. Feel and believe that your body has transformed into a body of the medicinal nectar that heals everything that you think, see, hear, and/or touch.

Finally, enjoy the feeling of peace and joy, joyful peace, the freedom from all impurities.

Then relax in open awareness of the peace and joy, joyful peace, in total silence, without grasping at it or needing to think in words about it.

5. *Transform Your Body into a Body of Blessing Light and Energy*

Think, feel, and believe that by the power of the blessing light of the Healing Buddhas, your body has transformed into a body of blessing light. Your body is no longer a body of gross elements, flesh and blood. It is a body of blessing light, amazingly bright, as if it were made of the light of billions of suns.

Your body has transformed into a body of blessing energy, heat and bliss, blissful heat. Your whole body, from the top of your head to the soles of your feet, is totally transformed into a body of blessing energies.

Finally, enjoy the stainless feeling and boundless power of your body.

Then be one with the feeling of peace and joy generated by the pure quality and boundless power of your body. Relax in open awareness of

Buddhist Meditations

peace and joy, joyful peace, in total silence, without grasping at it or analyzing it.

6. See That Your Body Is Made of Infinite Cells of Light and Energy

See that your body is a body made of billions and billions of cells. Each one is a blossoming cell of colorful light, as if made of rainbow light. They are individual cells, cells with individual structures and qualities. Each cell is blossoming with blessing light, bright and colorful light, like blossoming flowers of rainbow light.

Each cell is powerful, a cell of blessing energy, heat and bliss, blissful heat.

You can now repeat this exercise for each part of your body, as follows:

Your head is made of billions of cells, individual cells. Each cell is a cell of blessing light, bright and colorful. Each is a powerful cell, a cell of blessing energies, heat and bliss, blissful heat.

Your upper body is made of billions of cells, individual cells. Each cell is a cell of blessing light, bright and colorful. Each is a powerful cell, a cell of blessing energies, heat and bliss, blissful heat.

Your arms and hands are made of billions of cells, individual cells. Each cell is a cell of blessing light, bright and colorful. Each is a powerful cell, a cell of blessing energies, heat and bliss, blissful heat.

Your abdomen is made of billions of cells, individual cells. Each cell is a cell of blessing light, bright and colorful. Each is a powerful cell, a cell of blessing energies, heat and bliss, blissful heat.

Your legs and feet are made of billions of cells, individual cells. Each cell is a cell of blessing light, bright and colorful. Each is a powerful cell, a cell of blessing energies, heat and bliss, blissful heat.

Your body is a body of billions and billions of cells, individual cells. Each cell is a cell of blessing light, bright and colorful. See and feel the beauty and boundlessness of your body. Each cell is a powerful cell, a cell of blessing energies, heat and bliss, blissful heat.

Feel and believe that the blissful heat of the blessing energy has completely purified your physical toxins and mental impurities and that not even a trace of them has been left behind. Feel the total purity and cleanness of your body.

Finally, enjoy the feeling of the infinite nature of your body: the infinite cells, infinite purity, and infinite energies. Enjoy the peace and joy created by the infinite nature of your body.

Then relax in open awareness of peace and joy, joyful peace, in total silence, without grasping at it or needing to think in words about it.

7. Feel That Each Cell Is a Boundless Pure Land of Healing Buddhas

With your mind's eye, look at your forehead, between your eyebrows. There are hundreds of thousands of cells, cells of blessing light filled with blessing energy of blissful heat.

Now, choose one cell among those cells on your forehead. Then imagine that you are entering that cell, as if you were entering a room.

Think and feel that this cell is as vast as the universe. Feel the vastness and boundlessness of this cell, as if you had entered outer space. This cell has no end or boundary. Feel the clarity and beauty of this cell, as it is a cell of blessing light, colorful and radiant light. Feel the power and energy of this cell, as it is a cell made of blessing energy, blissful heat. Feel the peace and joy of this blessed cell, as all of it is translucent, calm, clear, colorful, and boundless.

With your mind's eye, see the Healing Buddha in the center of this vast cell of blessing light. His body is made of amazingly bright blue light, as if a mountain of lapis lazuli were touched by the light of thousands of suns.

On a huge blossoming lotus and moon seat, the radiant and youthful Healing Buddha is sitting in meditative posture. His body is a body of radiant light, like a mountain of lapis lazuli but made of light. He is dressed in three simple ascetic robes of light. With a supreme giving gesture, he holds a myrobalam (arura), the king of medicinal plants, in his right hand. With a contemplative gesture, he holds an ascetic's bowl filled with healing ambrosia in his left hand.

He is the embodiment of all the sources of blessing, the Buddhas, bodhisattvas, and sages.

He is full of love for each being and for you, as a mother for her only child. His enlightened mind sees everything simultaneously, as he sees with his omniscient wisdom. He has the power to heal all problems and grant all wishes, if you are open to this, for he is the pure nature and quality of the universe, the source of all well-being.

154

Feel the warmth in the presence of the Healing Buddha, just as you feel warmth, joy, and coziness when you sit by a fire in freezing weather.

Feel the total protection and relief of being in the care of the Healing Buddha, as if you were a baby alone in an empty room crying in fear and suddenly your parents walked in and gave you full attention and care.

Feel the total fulfillment of all your needs forever by having the omnipresent Healing Buddha as your protector, your companion, the source of blessings. Wealth, fame, power, and even physical health will end, but the presence of the inner Healing Buddha—the body of peace, joy, and wisdom—once found and preserved, will never end.

Now, think, feel, and believe that the Healing Buddha is surrounded by an infinite number of Healing Buddhas: Buddhas and bodhisattvas and sages in male and female forms, like the moon in the midst of an infinite number of stars and planets in a dark night sky.

All the Healing Buddhas are looking at you with eyes of compassion and omniscience that see everything simultaneously. They are all caring for you with the power to heal every ill.

Feel the warmth of being in the presence of the billions of Healing Buddhas. Feel the security of being in the care of the billions of Healing Buddhas. Feel the fulfillment of all your needs by having the billions of Healing Buddhas as your source of blessings.

So this cell is a pure land, a pure land of Healing Buddhas.

If you feel any pressure from excess energy, remember that this cell is made of light and that it is boundless and has no restrictions.

You can now deepen this meditation by extending it to other parts of your body, as follows:

Now, think again that your forehead is made of hundreds of thousands of cells, cells of blessing light. Each cell is a cell of blessing energy, blissful heat. Each is a vast pure land, a pure land of Healing Buddhas. In each pure land, there is the Healing Buddha surrounded by an infinite number of male and female Healing Buddhas.

Think and feel that your head is made of billions of cells, cells of blessing light. Each cell is a cell of blessing energy, blissful heat. Each is a vast pure land, a pure land of Healing Buddhas. In each pure land, there is the Healing Buddha surrounded by an infinite number of male and female Healing Buddhas.

155

Think and feel that your upper body is made of billions of cells, cells of blessing light. Each cell is a cell of blessing energy, blissful heat. Each is a vast pure land, a pure land of Healing Buddhas. In each pure land, there is the Healing Buddha surrounded by an infinite number of male and female Healing Buddhas.

Think and feel that your arms and hands are made of billions of cells, cells of blessing light. Each cell is a cell of blessing energy, blissful heat. Each is a vast pure land, a pure land of Healing Buddhas. In each pure land, there is the Healing Buddha surrounded by an infinite number of male and female Healing Buddhas.

Think and feel that your abdomen is made of billions of cells, cells of blessing light. Each cell is a cell of blessing energy, blissful heat. Each is a vast pure land, a pure land of Healing Buddhas. In each pure land, there is the Healing Buddha surrounded by an infinite number of male and female Healing Buddhas.

Think and feel that your legs and feet are made of billions of cells, cells of blessing light. Each cell is a cell of blessing energy, blissful heat. Each is a vast pure land, a pure land of Healing Buddhas. In each pure land, there is the Healing Buddha surrounded by an infinite number of male and female Healing Buddhas.

Think and feel that your body, your whole body, is made of billions and billions of cells, cells of blessing light. Each cell is a cell of blessing energy, blissful heat. Each is a vast pure land, a pure land of infinite Healing Buddhas. In each pure land, there is the Healing Buddha surrounded by an infinite number of male and female Healing Buddhas.

Think about the infinite array of pure lands and Buddhas of your miraculous sacred body. Feel that every pure land is a world of light, beauty, peace, and joy. Every Buddha is a Buddha of omnipresent love and power and omniscient wisdom.

Feel the experience of amazing warmth, absolute security, total fulfillment, ultimate peace, great joy, and boundless openness in yourself in the presence of the Healing Buddha.

Finally, enjoy the feeling of your body's being billions and billions of pure lands adorned with oceans of Buddhas. Enjoy the feeling of peace and joy of being the boundless pure lands with infinite Healing Buddhas.

Then relax in open awareness of the feeling of boundless and infinite peace and joy, joyful peace, in total silence, without grasping at it or thinking about it.

Note: After gaining good experience with this meditation, if you wish, you can explore the following imagery as part of the meditation:

Think and feel that each of the infinite numbers of Buddhas of your body is a body of billions of boundless cells of light. Each cell of their bodies is a pure land made of light and blessing energy. Each of these pure lands has a Healing Buddha surrounded by an infinite number of male and female Healing Buddhas.

Then you can again think and feel that each of those infinite numbers of Buddhas in the cells of the Buddha bodies also has a body of billions of boundless cells of light. Each cell is a pure land of light and blessing energy. In each of these pure lands, there is a Healing Buddha surrounded by an infinite number of male and female Healing Buddhas.

All the Buddhas are gathered in infinite assemblies of great peace and joy.

You can think and feel yourself into more limitless visions and feelings of the Buddhas and pure lands.

Note that it is important to have good experience with the first seven stages of meditation before you proceed to the next stage, healing with the waves of blessing light and energy.

8.   Heal with the Waves of Blessing Light and Energy

Think and feel that you are breathing air. You are breathing in and breathing out, in and out, in and out. You are breathing from the stomach through the respiratory channels, in and out, in and out. See and feel the breathing in and breathing out.

Now think that you are not just breathing in and out from the stomach through the respiratory channels but that every cell of your body is breathing. All the cells are breathing in and breathing out, breathing in and out, in and out.

Every cell of your body, from the top of your head to the soles of your feet, is breathing, breathing in and breathing out, in and out.

Now think and feel that your breathing is not just the breathing of air but that your breathing is the waves of blessing energy, heat and bliss, and blessing light. Like the waves of the ocean, your breathing has taken the form of waves of light and energy, blissful heat.

When you exhale, think and feel that every Healing Buddha in every pure land of your body is sending waves of blessing light and energy as offerings to all the other Buddhas in every pure land of your body.

When you inhale, think and feel that every Healing Buddha in every pure land of your body is receiving and enjoying the gift of waves of blessing light and energy from all the other Buddhas in every pure land of your body.

Send healing waves out and receive healing waves in. Send out and receive in. Out and in.

Feel and enjoy the sending and receiving of the waves of blessing light and energy by the infinite number of Buddhas of your boundless body. Feel the increase of heat and blissful energy of your body.

Think and feel that every Buddha of every pure land of your body, from the top of your head to the soles of your feet, is actively sharing and enjoying the waves of blessing light and the energy of blissful heat.

Think and feel that all the Buddhas of every pure land of your body, from the top of your head to the soles of your feet, are harmoniously functioning as one team, actively sharing the waves of blessing light and blessing energy.

Every Buddha of every pure land is connected with all the others in the current of blessing waves of light and energy, blissful heat.

The healing light and energy increase in every Buddha of every pure land as the blessing waves move with your breathing through your body.

As the blessing light and energy increase in every Buddha, more and more powerful lights and energies radiate from them, infusing your whole universelike body with all-pervasive blessing energies.

Feel that the amazing power of the energy is flowing through your body, filling your whole body, from the top of your head to the soles of your feet.

Now briefly think of and feel how your sensitive mind usually clings to the notion of "I," "me," and "my." Think, feel, and believe that the waves of blessing light and energy have melted down and evaporated all the thoughts, feelings, and sensitivities of "I," "me," and "my," as ice melts in the summer sun. Your woundlike "I," "me," and "my" have totally vanished. Now there is nothing to be protected, nothing about which to feel insecure, sensitive, or unfulfilled, since "I," "me," and "my" themselves have completely disappeared without a trace. Feel peace and joy, unconditional joyful peace.

Again, think, feel, and believe that your body is not just filled with pure lands and Buddhas but that it is a body of boundless blessing light, infinite pure lands, and limitless Buddhas.

See and feel the boundless peace and joy of your sacred body.

Finally, enjoy the amazingly powerful waves of boundless blessing energy. Enjoy the waves of blissful heat moving through all the infinite pure lands and Buddhas of your body. Enjoy the boundless blissful heat.

Then relax in open awareness of boundless blissful heat, in total silence, without grasping at it or analyzing it.

Note: You can also add one or both of the following to this meditation:

To Heal a Particular Problem. If you are experiencing a particular problem that you wish to heal, you can meditate thus:

See and feel every cell of your body as a body of pure lands and Healing Buddhas. But at the location where you are experiencing your particular problem or problems, there is an island in ordinary form, a collection of sick cells. Now visualize that your problem—it could be sickness, sadness, collected poisons, hardened tumors, fixations on unresolved emotions, or unhealed wounds—has taken the form of a dark cloud, filth, ice, flame, or pain. Then think that this form is emitting the sensation of your problem and feel it briefly.

Then think, feel, and believe that blessing lights and energy waves are coming from every Healing Buddha of every pure land of your body. These waves of light and blissful heat energy are touching, pacifying, and dissolving the image and feeling of your problem. Feel and believe that the problems you were experiencing have now completely gone. They have vanished forever without leaving any trace. Enjoy the freedom from those problems for a while.

To Further Deepen Your Meditation. After gaining good experience with the meditation given in the first eight stages, you could deepen your meditation even further by adding the following:

Think and feel that each of the infinite numbers of Healing Buddhas of your body is made of billions of cells of blessing light.

Each cell of their bodies is a pure land filled with an infinite number of Buddhas. Each Buddha is sending and receiving blessing lights with energy waves.

Again, each of those infinite Healing Buddhas is made of billions of cells of blessing light. Each cell is a pure land filled with an infinite number of Buddhas. Each Buddha is sending and receiving blessing lights with energy waves.

See, feel, and believe that your body is a body of an infinite cycle of healing. Your body is a body of infinite boundless pure lands of beauty and joy. Your body is a body of infinite Healing Buddhas with love and wisdom. Your body is a body of infinite waves of blessing lights and blissful heat energy.

Note: If you have any proliferating sick cells and wish to do so, you can combine this meditation with the optional meditation given in Chapter 6, exercise 7: "Perform a Special Meditation to Heal Proliferating Sick Cells" (page 95).

9. Sing AH, the Sound of Blessing Light and Energy Waves

The sound AH is the soothing sound of the waves of blessing light and blessing energy. In harmony with the waves of blessing light and energy, repeatedly sing AH and hear the sound of AH—slowly and continuously.

Sing AH in three tones of voice:

1. First, in a loud and inspiring voice, sing AH, the sound of healing light and healing energy, blissful heat.

    Sing while you are exhaling. Think and feel that all the Healing Buddhas of your body, with love, are sending offerings of the AH sound with healing light and energy waves to all the other Healing Buddhas of your body, from the top of your head to the soles of your feet.

    While inhaling, just hear the singing sound of AH. Think and feel that every Healing Buddha of your body, with joy, is receiving the soothing singing vibration of AH, the sound of healing light and energy waves. Every Healing Buddha is receiving the gift of AH from every other Healing Buddha of your body, from the top of your head to the soles of your feet.

    Exhaling, sing AH, the soothing sound of the waves of healing light and energy sent by the Healing Buddhas. Inhaling, hear the sound of AH, the sound of the waves of healing light and energy.

    Think and feel that all the Healing Buddhas of your body, from the top of your head to the soles of your feet, are enjoying the sound of AH, the sound of blessing waves, like the sound of a great symphony.

Think and feel that the sound of AH is invoking all the Healing Buddhas to send streams of blessing lights with healing energy and AH.

The powerful, joyous sound of AH completely fills all the pure lands of your whole body with waves of radiant light and boundless, blissful heat.

2. Then, in a soft voice, as if you were almost whispering, sing AH, the sound of the waves of healing light and healing energy, blissful heat.

While exhaling, sing AH softly and think and feel that every Healing Buddha of your body, with love, is sending waves of the singing sound of AH, the sound of healing light and energy, as an offering to all the other Healing Buddhas of your body.

While inhaling, just hear the singing sound of AH and think and feel that every Healing Buddha of your body, with joy, is receiving the singing sound of AH, the sound of the healing light and energy waves, as a gift from all the other Healing Buddhas of your body.

Every Healing Buddha of your body, from the top of your head to the soles of your feet, is enjoying AH, the sound of blessing light and blissful heat waves.

3. Then, in the voice of the mind, silently sing the sound of AH, the sound of the waves of blessing light and blessing energy, the blissful heat of the Healing Buddhas.

While exhaling and inhaling, sing the sound of AH and think and feel that every Healing Buddha of your body, with love, is sending to all the other Healing Buddhas of your body and receiving from all the other Healing Buddhas the offering of the singing sound of AH, the sound of the waves of healing light and energy.

Hear and feel AH, the sound of blessing energy waves that is powerfully resonating in every pure land and in every Healing Buddha, like the powerful sound of every wave of the ocean.

Think and feel that AH, the sound of the blessing energy waves of the Healing Buddhas, is boundlessly bursting out of every pore of your body and into the atmosphere, like sounds resonating through a wall.

Finally, enjoy the nature of AH, the boundless blessing sound and energy waves, as they generate boundless waves of blissful heat and light.

Then relax in open awareness of the nature of the blessing sound waves of AH, in total silence, without grasping at it or analyzing it.

Note: The following exercises are variations on this stage of the meditation:

- Exhaling, think and feel that every Healing Buddha of your body is sending out waves of AH, which fill all the pure lands with a blessed cloud of energy, light, and blissful heat, as a greenhouse is filled with the scent of flowers.

  Inhaling, think and feel that each pure land and every Healing Buddha is filling up with a blessed cloud of energy, light, and blissful heat, as a greenhouse is filled with the scent of flowers.

- After gaining good experience with the sound of AH, think and feel that each of the infinite numbers of healing Buddhas of your body is made of billions of cells of light. Each cell of their bodies is a pure land filled with infinite Healing Buddhas. Each Healing Buddha is sending and receiving blessing sound waves of AH and blessing light and energy waves.

  Again, each of those infinite Healing Buddhas within the Buddhas is made of billions of light cells. Each cell is a pure land filled with infinite Healing Buddhas. Each of those Healing Buddhas is sending and receiving blessing sound waves of AH and blessing light and energy waves.

  You can think and feel yourself further and deeper into a limitless scope of meditation.

10. Perform the Blossoming Lotus Movement with Blessing Waves

Fold the palms of your hands together at your heart, like a flower bud. Think that your fingers and hands are fingers and hands of billions of pure lands, pure lands of light. Every pure land is vast and boundless as the sky. Every boundless pure land is filled with billions of Healing Buddhas, Healing Buddhas of love, wisdom, and power. Every pure land and every Healing Buddha is made of blessing light with blissful heat.

As you breathe, think, feel, and believe that all the Healing Buddhas are breathing, breathing in the form of blessing energy, blissful heat. They are sending and receiving waves of blessing energy with the sound of AH.

As your hands join together in the form of a flower bud, think and feel that all the cells of your fingers and hands are touching one another, as the petals and pistils of a flower are in close touch with one another.

Now open your palms in utmost slow motion, as if they were hardly moving. Move your hands apart sideways, about six to eight inches, with your hands close beside your body at shoulder level.

While moving your hands, feel every subtle movement that is taking place in your hands. Feel that your hand movements are instigating chain reactions of blessing energy. Feel the sensation of a blessing energy current flowing through every pure land and every Healing Buddha in your fingers and hands, like the flow of a river.

As the pure lands and Healing Buddhas of your hands are being stimulated with the flow of energy currents, think and feel that your hands are blossoming with bright light and blissful heat, as a dewy flower blossoms in full, bright sunlight.

The following passages repeat the same awareness movements of touching and opening but in different parts of your body:

Slowly bring your palms back together and feel that the blessing energies of every pure land and every Healing Buddha of your arms are making contact and joining with one another. Feel the energy current that connects the pure lands and Healing Buddhas of your arms to one another.

Then, open your palms in utmost slow motion, as if they were hardly moving. Think and feel that the movement of opening your hands is activating blessing energy waves in every pure land and every Healing Buddha of your arms. Think and feel that all the pure lands and Healing Buddhas of your arms are opening like a blossoming flower.

Slowly bringing your palms back together, feel that the blessing energies of all the pure lands and Buddhas of your upper body are making contact and joining with one another. Feel the energy current from the joining and touching of all the pure lands and Buddhas of your upper body.

Then, open your palms in utmost slow motion, as if they were hardly moving. Think and feel that the movement of opening your hands is activating waves of healing energy that flows like a current through all the pure lands and Buddhas of your upper body.

Again, slowly bringing your palms back together, feel that the blessing energies of every pure land and every Buddha of your head

163

Meditations on the Healing Buddha

are making contact and joining with one another. Feel the energy current from the joining and touching of the blessing energies of all the pure lands and Buddhas of your head.

Then, open your palms in utmost slow motion, as if they were hardly moving. Think and feel that the movement of opening your hands is activating waves of healing energy that flows like a current through all the pure lands and Buddhas of your head.

Again, slowly bringing your palms back together, feel that the blessing energies of all the pure lands and Buddhas of your abdomen are making contact and joining with one another. Feel the energy current from the joining and touching of the blessing energies of all the pure lands and Buddhas of your abdomen.

Then, open your palms in utmost slow motion, as if they were hardly moving. Think and feel that the movement of opening your hands is activating waves of healing energy that flows like a current through all the pure lands and Buddhas of your abdomen.

Again, slowly bringing your palms back together, feel that the blessing energies of all the pure lands and Buddhas of your legs and feet are making contact and joining with one another. Feel the energy current from the joining and touching of the blessing energies of all the pure lands and Buddhas of your legs and feet.

Then, open your palms in utmost slow motion, as if they were hardly moving. Think and feel that the movement of opening your hands is activating waves of healing energy that flows like a current through all the pure lands and Buddhas of your legs and feet.

Finally, enjoy the movements of the blessing energy currents through every pure land and Healing Buddha of your body. Enjoy the boundless, blissful heat of the movements.

Then, just relax in the open awareness of the boundless power of the energy currents, in total silence, without grasping at your experience or needing to think in words about it.

Note: Here are some ways to broaden this stage of the meditation and incorporate its power into your everyday activities:

- After gaining a deeper experience with this exercise, you could broaden this meditation with movement by visualizing even more elaborate imagery, as follows:

    Think and feel that each of the infinite numbers of Healing

Buddhas of your body is made of billions of cells of light. Each cell of their bodies is a pure land filled with infinite Healing Buddhas. As you slowly move, great blessing waves and the sound of AH move through each of those pure lands and Healing Buddhas.

Again, each of those infinite Healing Buddhas within the Buddhas is made of billions of cells of light. Each cell is a pure land filled with infinite Healing Buddhas. With each movement, each pure land and each Healing Buddha is filled with great blessing energy waves and the sound of AH.

• Gradually, you could incorporate the awareness of movement into most of your everyday activities to feel the flow or current of blessing energies in your body.

You could create the harmonious movement of blessing energies in your body by standing and rocking your body from right to left, by stretching your muscles and relaxing them, by walking, by slow dancing, by doing yoga exercises, and finally, even by running.

You can repeat the awareness movements of any part of your body as many times as you like and also incorporate the singing sound of AH into the waves of movements.

PERFORM OTHER HEALING MOVEMENTS THAT BRING BLESSINGS (OPTIONAL)

Immerse yourself in the awareness of the blessing energies of your body, with its boundless pure lands and infinite Buddhas. Bathe in the feeling of the blessing energies. Be aware of the waves of blessing energies moving through your body, with its boundless pure lands and infinite Buddhas.

Then do any one of the following healing movements or do all of them one after another. These exercises can be done in any position that is comfortable, such as lying down or standing.

Stretching and Relaxing. Very slowly stretch your body, the joints and muscles, for a minute or two. Stretch the upper part of your body upward and the lower part of your body downward, like a tree reaching toward the sky while its roots grow into the earth. With total awareness, feel the blessing energy being generated by the slow, subtle movement.

Feel that the movement is activating chain reactions of blessing energy, blissful heat, that flows like a current through the boundless pure

Meditations on the Healing Buddha

lands of every cell of your body. Bring your awareness to any particular problem—for example, any injured or blocked area—and feel the flow of energy bringing the maximum amount of healing to this area. Feel and believe that the infinite Buddhas in every pure land are sending out their blessings with the movements and that they are rejoicing in the healing of your body. Continue this stretch for a minute or so, however long is comfortable.

Then relax your body. Take a minute or so to do this, allowing the joints and muscles to move back into place. Feel the blissful heat of the healing energy moving and flowing through the boundless pure lands with their infinite Buddhas. These enlightened ones are receiving and celebrating the healing energy from every other Buddha. Healing blessings are overflowing in every one of the boundless pure lands.

Slowly repeat the same stretching and relaxing of your body. Be aware of the feelings of the subtle movements of stretching and relaxing. Rejoice in the feeling of blessings being sent out and received by the loving Buddhas in their pure lands.

Note that the movements of all these exercises should be done with very relaxed breathing. In whatever way you find comfortable, you could synchronize your inhalation and exhalation with the movements.

You could also do a similar exercise by lying on your back and performing a very slow bicycle-pedaling motion with your feet.

Expanding Your Body as You Breathe. With total awareness, very slowly expand your whole body—the organs, muscles, and nerves—while inhaling. Then relax your body—the organs, muscles, and nerves—while exhaling. Be aware of your subtle movements as you expand and relax your body. Feel that the movement is activating a chain reaction of blessings that flow through the boundless pure lands and infinite Buddhas of your body. During this and all the healing movements, focus your awareness particularly on any problem areas. Feel that the blessings are completely healing the problem.

Rejoice in the flow of energy through all the pure lands of your body. Slowly repeat the expansion and relaxation of your body again and again.

Tightening and Relaxing. With total awareness, very slowly tighten the muscles of your body for a minute or two. Then relax the muscles for a minute or two. Be aware of the very subtle movements of tightening followed by relaxing. The tightening and relaxing are so subtle that the movements may or may not even be visible but are felt at the energy level.

Feel that each movement is activating an outpouring of blessings shared by the infinite Buddhas of your body and that this blessed energy is flowing like a river or current through your boundless pure lands. Slowly repeat the tightening and relaxing of your body over and over again.

Swaying Your Body. Sway with a very subtle movement, to one side for a minute or so and then to the other. Although this movement might be imperceptible to anyone who was looking at you, your mind and body feel that the movement is activating powerful chain reactions of healing energy. The energy is flowing through the boundless pure lands of your body with its infinite Buddhas. Each Buddha is sharing its blessings of warmth, love, and joy with every other enlightened one throughout your boundless body. Repeat the swaying of your body to the left and to the right again and again and rejoice in the abundance of blessings.

Finally, when you have completed any one or all of the exercises, relax in oneness with the results of your meditation, without grasping at it or needing to think in words about it.

11. Share the Blessing Waves with the Whole Universe

Now think and feel that each of the infinite pure lands and Healing Buddhas of your body is sending beams of blessing light with waves of blessing energy and the sound of AH as offerings in all directions.

Think and feel that beams of blessing light and blessing energy with the sound of AH have filled the bodies of every being and the whole universe. By the mere touch of blessing energies, all the confusion, sadness, and pain of beings are dispelled. The whole universe is transformed into a pure land of blessing light and energy. The suffering of all beings is dispelled, and their gross forms are transformed into bodies of blessing light filled with blissful heat. All beings are celebrating in a mighty chorus of AH.

Every cell of every being is transformed into a pure land with numerous Healing Buddhas. Every atom of the earth is transformed into a pure land filled with an infinite number of Healing Buddhas.

All the pure lands and Buddhas are sharing with one another the

167

waves of blessing light and blessing energy with joyous sounds of AH. The whole universe has become one, in a cycle of Healing Buddha blessings.

The whole universe is filled with beams of blessing light, waves of blessing energy, and the celebratory sound of AH. The whole of existence before you is transformed into amazing pure lands filled with infinite Healing Buddhas.

Finally, enjoy the universal peace and joy generated by this sharing of healing blessing with all.

Then relax in open awareness of universal peace and joy, joyful peace, without grasping at it or needing to think in words about it.

Note: If you feel concerned about being exposed to external harm by opening yourself to the whole universe, you could supplement your sharing of blessing waves with the whole universe by using the optional meditation presented in Chapter 6, exercise 11: "Protect Yourself with a Healing Aura" (page 112).

12. *Rest in Oneness with the Healing Experience*

Recognize the positive experience that you have generated as the result of this healing meditation session. It could be the feeling of peace, joy, bliss, spaciousness, power, richness, oneness, or any positive feeling.

If you have many positive experiences, choose the most prominent or the one that you feel is most beneficial for your need. After recognizing the experience, just enjoy that particular experience. Enjoy the feeling of that experience, again and again.

Now let your mind merge with that experience and be one with it, like water being poured into water. You and your healing experience are merged as one. You and your healing experience have become one, the feeling in the feeling. Relax in the feeling without grasping at it or needing to think about it in words or concepts.

Relax in open awareness of the experience; be at one with it, without grasping.

Again and again, go back to the state of oneness with whatever you are feeling. Rest in the feeling. Relax in it. Relax openly in oneness with joy and peace. Rest in joyful peace.

Note: Don't try to shape or create an experience in one way or another. Don't have any expectation of succeeding or any fear of failing.

Just let it be as it is. This is the way to find your center. This is the way to sow the seed of healing at a deeper level in your mind. When you can find and maintain your own inner qualities, there is no need to look for any other source of healing.

DEDICATION, ASPIRATION, AND BENEDICTION

If you are practicing Buddhism, it will be good after completing your meditation to take some time for a dedication and blessing, as follows:

Dedication. From the depth of your mind, with great joy, offer and dedicate all the merits that you have to all beings as the means of healing their sufferings, with no expectation of reward for yourself in return.

If you dedicate your merits to infinite beings, the merits increase to infinitude instead of decreasing. Feel the great joy of being able to offer all your merits to others.

Aspiration. With that dedication, make aspirations by thinking (and saying):

> By the power of the infinite Healing Buddhas and the boundless pure lands, by the power of the meditations that I have done, and by the power of the merits that I have accumulated, may all beings have happiness, peace, and joy.
>
> May the mental and physical pains and sufferings of all beings cease. May the blessing light and blessing energy of the Healing Buddhas always be with every being and never apart or separate from them. May every being swiftly attain the ultimate peace and joy, full enlightenment. May the whole universe enjoy great peace and joy, the prosperity of the Buddha pure lands.
>
> May I always be with the blessing light and blessing power of the Healing Buddhas without separation, day and night, awake or asleep, in good times and bad, life after life, until the attainment of buddhahood. May I always be the source of blessing light and blessing energy, peace and joy, for the whole universe.

Benediction. Think that all the Buddhas in the sky and in your body are conferring upon you, in one thunderous voice, the following benedictions:

May all your prayers be answered. May all your wishes be fulfilled.
. . . May your [particular problems] be fully healed, leaving no trace
behind. May you always be with the blessing light and blessing
energy of the Healing Buddhas without separation. May you always be the source of blessing light and blessing energy for all
beings and for the whole universe.

Note: With the merits as the seed, whatever aspirations you make will
come to fruition. The Buddha said:

> All happenings [arise] according to the conditions.
> Conditions are based on mental attitudes.
> Whoever makes any aspiration,
> He or she achieves the result accordingly.[8]

THE HEALING BUDDHA
MEDITATION IN BRIEF

Start by devoting your time and energy to the first stage of meditation.
When you have gained some experience with this stage, then you can
add the next stage to it.

When you feel that a particular stage of the meditation is bringing
greater peace, joy, and stability, you are ready to add the next exercise.
If you are experiencing uneasiness with a particular stage, then you
need to wait before adding the next exercise. Also, you can do this
healing meditation series with or without stages 9 and 10 (the sound
of AH and the healing movements).

Once you are familiar with all the exercises, you can meditate on
all twelve stages in every meditation session.

When you become proficient in these twelve exercises, you may
wish to abbreviate the time of meditation. A brief version is as follows:

First, take a couple of deep breaths and release all tensions and
strains with the outgoing breath. Feel the calmness in your body, from
the top of your head to the soles of your feet.

Think, "I am going to meditate on the Healing Buddha to bring
healing blessings for the sake of all beings."

Visualize, feel, and believe in the presence of the actual Healing
Buddha in the sky before you.

Pray with strong devotion to the Healing Buddha. Receive the

Buddhist Meditations

blessings in the form of light (or nectar) with blessing energy, heat, and bliss.

Think and feel that your body is purified. Then think and feel that it is transformed into a body of blessing light and energy.

See that your body is made of billions of cells. Each is a cell of light, vast as the universe and filled with blessing energy, blissful heat. Your body has become a body of light and blissful heat. Feel the purity and power of boundless energy.

See that each cell is a pure land in which are dwelling the Healing Buddha and an ocean of enlightened ones in male and female forms. All are enjoying the healing celebration, singing and dancing in graceful movements.

When you exhale, feel that every Healing Buddha of your body is sending blessing energy waves as offerings to all the other Buddhas. When you inhale, feel that all the Healing Buddhas are receiving the blessing energy waves as gifts from all the other Buddhas.

All the Buddhas are active, and all are linked with one another in the current of the blessing energy waves. Feel the wholeness and harmony of your body as the great waves of blessing energies move through it.

Then share the healing energy waves with all beings and the whole universe. Transform the universe and every being into blessing light and blessing energy.

Recognize and enjoy the result of the meditation. Relax in open awareness of the feeling without grasping at it or needing to think in words about it.

Finally, dedicate all the merits of the meditation to healing all the mother beings and the whole universe.

Note: If you prefer, you could condense your meditation session by focusing only on key stages:

Begin by bringing your mind back to your body (exercise 1).

Then, focus on seeing that your body is made of infinite cells of light and energy (exercise 6), feeling that each cell is a boundless pure land of Healing Buddhas (exercise 7), and healing with the waves of blessing light and energy (exercise 8).

Finally, end by sharing the blessing waves with the universe (exercise 11) and resting in oneness with the healing experience (exercise 12).

Meditations on the Healing Buddha

9

HEALING MEDITATIONS FOR THE DYING AND DEAD

DEATH CAN BE A FEARFUL TIME, because we are leaving behind our bodies and everything else that we know. But it can also be a time of opportunity. Even though pain and fear may be part of death, dying can also be a period of great opening and peace, and even enlightenment.[1]

Buddhists believe that death and dying are ripe with possibility. The bardo, as Tibetan Buddhists call the transition between life and death, is a highly charged time when we greatly need healing. For the dying and dead, healing meditation can be very helpful.

Actually, there are a number of bardos, or transitional states. Life itself can be seen as a bardo, since it is the transition between birth and death. The best preparation for the great bardo of dying is to develop a peaceful mind in this life. Then, when the body dissolves at death, we will be ready.

If we have cultivated positive and peaceful habits of mind while we are alive, then we will take these habits or cyclic causations (karma) into death and any future life to which we may be born. Even for those who are not Buddhists or do not believe in reincarnation, developing a peaceful mind in this life can make death easier and more peaceful. At the time of death, when our minds are vulnerable and open, meditation and prayer can help us tremendously.

Meditation that uses the four healing powers can be our source of strength at death, just as it is while we are alive. We see images of peace, joy, and openness. We hear sounds and words as being peaceful, joyous, and celebratory. We open ourselves to peaceful and blissful feelings. And we believe in the healing power of these positive images, sounds, and feelings.

If our minds are positive and peaceful because of meditation, we can transform negative experiences into positive ones. Then, at the time of our death and during our travels through the bardo, our mental visions will arise as peaceful, loving, and powerful images. We will hear sounds as soothing and celebratory. We will feel peaceful and joyful experiences.

Such experiences will change the whole course and atmosphere of the journey through death from the darkness of confusion to the light of wisdom, from fear and sadness to confidence and joy, from the burning of negative emotions to the celebration of peace and joy, and from the rigidity of conceptual confinement to the openness of liberation.

Of course, if we are ordinary, struggling people, then sickness and death can be very difficult. It will help us to have family or friends to hold our hands, talk to us with soothing words, and pray with us. Even if we are lonely or frightened, we should feel confident that the best approach to dying is to relax the grasping quality of our minds as much as we can. Even if we are struggling with death, eventually we may be able to let go of grasping. The more we can do this, the better. In dying, we can discover more clearly than ever what letting go means. This can give us the peace we wish for.

If we are helping a sick or dying person, we should be honest, open, and natural with him or her. The most important thing is to find out what the person needs and not try to force our views or emotions upon him or her. Allow the sick or dying person to express himself or herself, including any worries and fears. Simply being there with the person, in a loving and supportive way, can be a wonderful consolation.

A BUDDHIST APPROACH TO DYING

Is the traditional Buddhist training on death beneficial and applicable for non-Buddhists?

Some people are open to Buddhist views on dying and death, even if they are not Buddhists. Others appreciate Buddhism but cannot easily accept Buddhist imagery and the complex views about death and what lies beyond. Finally, there are those who are totally closed to Buddhism and Buddhist ideas about death.

Some teachers think that if the dying person disliked or resisted Buddhist images and concepts during life, he or she may hold on to the same tendencies in the bardo, for habit-driven attitudes are not easily overcome. If that is the case, introducing Buddhist prayers could harm the person by causing confusion, dislike, or even hatred.

Other teachers think that it is beneficial to perform Buddhist death ceremonies for anyone who is dying or who is in the bardo. We could approach the person gently and introduce him or her to Buddhist enlightened images and prayers, even if the dying person wasn't open to Buddhism in his or her lifetime. The reason this could help is that those who are in the bardo will appreciate any peaceful, joyful, and powerful images and sounds. They will eagerly be seeking a shelter and relief. We could help them greatly or at least cause them no harm.

This second view may be true. However, as the bardo of dying is a very crucial juncture, it's probably best to play it absolutely safe. If you have doubts about using a traditional Buddhist approach to dying, with its unique imagery, it may be preferable to use a more universal approach, which I describe in the next section.

MEDITATIONS FOR THE DEAD OR DYING

If the dying person is a practicing Buddhist, you as a helper could do dharma meditation and say prayers as the person is dying and for forty-nine days after his or her death.

In many Tibetan Buddhist traditions, elaborate ceremonies are performed for the dead. With prayers to the Buddhas, you bring back the consciousness of the dead to the body or to an effigy. Then you perform detailed ceremonies intended to teach and instruct the dead person. You perform purifications and accumulate merits. Finally, you transfer the consciousness of the dead person into the mind of the Buddha and/or into a pure land.

As a helper, however, you should do whatever is feasible and beneficial. Instead of trying to do many things, the most beneficial approach will be to do the meditations and say the prayers that both you and the dying person are familiar with and do well.

Use those prayers and meditations to awaken the thought and feeling of the presence of the powerful Healing Buddhas to protect the person and lead him or her through the death process. Think and feel that you are both in the atmosphere of everlasting awareness of peace, joy, strength, and light and relax in those feelings. If the dying person can collaborate with you in these meditations, that will be beneficial. The prayers can be said aloud or silently.

If the person is not open to Buddhism, the following might be the best and safest approach. It is based on Buddhist principles, but it has the quality of universality that has been used in this book. So you could perform the following prayers and meditations for the dying or dead person:

1. Above in the sky, see many enlightened or heavenly beings, saints, or divinities made of light, infinite light. They are beings of great love, amazing peace, and total openness.
2. Hear the singing sound of AH, the universal sound, or any peaceful word or sound. Hear and feel boundless love, amazing peace, and total openness resounding as the sound of AH.
3. Then think of the dying person and feel his or her presence. Feel that this person is also seeing the presence of these beings of light, hearing the sound of AH, and feeling their boundless love, amazing peace, and total openness.
4. See and feel that the enlightened beings are sending their love, blessing, and power in the form of beams of light—warm, joyful, and powerful light—to the dying person. His or her whole body is filled with the blessing light. The mere touch of the blessing light pacifies all the anxieties, fear, confusion, and pain in this person and fills him or her with peace, joy, strength, and wisdom.
5. Feel that this person and you, as well as all the atmosphere surrounding you, are transformed into a world of light and feel as though you were both bathing in utmost peace and joy. Rest and relax in that feeling.

175

INSTRUCTIONS FOR THE DEAD OR DYING

If the dead or dying person is a Buddhist, or open to prayers and help, you can also talk to the person and send him or her positive messages, either aloud or in your thoughts:

- In the bardo, you might see wrathful, ugly, or frightening images. If you do, you must remember that these terrifying images are not real; they are creations and reflections of your own mind. They are mere images fabricated by your mind, like hallucinations or magic displays. Now you must think of them as images of light. Remember that they are peaceful, joyful, and open in their true nature and true quality. See them with openness as peaceful and joyful images.
- In the bardo, you might hear thundering sounds and frightening words. If you do, you must remember that these are mere creations of your mind. They are simply sounds fabricated by your mind, like hallucinations or echoes. Now you must remember that all sounds are peaceful and inspiring in their true nature and true quality. Hear the sounds joyfully as peaceful sounds.
- In the bardo, you might feel unpleasant, lonely, and fearful sensations. If you do, you must remember that these sensations are merely created by your own mind, fabricated like hallucinations or nightmares. You must remember that all thoughts and feelings are peaceful and joyful in their true nature and true quality. Feel your thoughts and sensations as joyful and peaceful.
- Do not get attached to the images, sounds, or sensations, grasp at them, or be frightened by them. See the images openly, hear the sounds peacefully, and feel the experiences joyfully. They are the images, sounds, and feelings of the true nature and qualities of your own mind.

If the person is open to Buddhism, explain to him or her how to visualize the image of the Healing Buddha (or any familiar Buddha image) accompanied by hosts of compassionate male and female beings of light. Gently tell the person the following:

See these fully enlightened beings as overflowing with love, peace, joy, power, and wisdom. They are present in the sky before you to protect you and lead you on your journey. They are here to support you.

Hear all sound as the sound of the loving voices of the enlightened ones. Hear all sound as the sound of prayers (or the sound of AH), sounds that are totally peaceful, open, and joyful.

Feel the presence of the Healing Buddhas, the enlightened ones. Feel boundless peace and joy in their presence. Feel the warmth of their presence. Feel the security of their presence. Feel the fulfillment of all your needs in their presence. Feel and believe that from now on, you are protected and guided by the enlightened beings.

HOW HELPERS AND SURVIVORS SHOULD BEHAVE

Those helping the dead and dying should offer spiritual assistance according to the experience in Buddhist meditation of both the helper and the person being helped. Specifically:

- If the dying person is open to help but is unfamiliar with meditation and the helper is better trained, then the helper must say prayers, perform ceremonies, and give instructions on death out loud to the dying person. The instructions should be brief, clear, simple, and heartfelt.

    It is important that the helper place the main emphasis on his or her own meditative experience. In this way, the helper may be able to lead the dying person through the process of dying and the bardo and reach the peaceful and joyful shore, like carrying a sick person across a torrent.

- If the dying person is a well-trained meditator but not a highly accomplished one and is more or less equal to the helper, then the helper should say prayers, perform ceremonies, and remind the person of the instructions on dying.

    It is important for the helper to think and feel that he or she and the dying person are uniting in the meditation. This approach can help the dying person, like crossing a torrent together holding hands for support.

- If the dying person is a highly accomplished meditator, more skilled than the helper, then the helper can remain in contemplative meditation and say prayers but quietly or at a distance.

Here the important point is to let the dying person go at his or her own pace. The helper should not touch the body of the accomplished meditator. If possible, no sound should be made as long as this person is in the final stages of dying. Through touch, sound, or suggestions, an ordinary person could distract the accomplished meditator from his or her journey. Only when the process of death is complete should the helper say prayers and perform death rituals aloud in the presence of the body.

The age-old Tibetan rituals for the dying and dead call upon those who are living to meditate and pray. Prayers and meditations can lead the dead person directly to spiritual attainment. But even if they do not, they will create meritorious karma for the dead person and help to improve his or her future lives.

If we have solid experience of meditation and the four healing powers of mind, we will be able to offer great support to others at the time of their death. By offering our help to others, we ourselves will be sustained by the healing energies of peace and joy. We will also joyfully welcome our own death when it comes. Healing is not meant just for the body. We can heal the mind and life itself, this life and the afterlife, ourselves and others, now and forever.

Buddhist Meditations

Appendix 1

BUDDHIST SOURCES OF THE
HEALING MEDITATIONS

The Healing Power of Mind, this book's predecessor, was received with great appreciation by Buddhists and non-Buddhists alike, beyond anything I had expected. However, some Buddhist scholars thought the first book contained materials that belonged to the New Age movement, whereas others felt it contained esoteric (Tantric) teachings that shouldn't have been included in a popular healing book.

To address these concerns, I would like to document the sources for the healing meditations, which are based on principles found in common (sutric) Buddhism.

Actually, the inspiration to write the book first came to me from my background as a practitioner of esoteric Buddhism. Only initiated trainees can practice esoteric meditations. But as I will make clear, many of the major points about healing are found in both common and esoteric teachings. In my books about healing, I have only used healing meditations that could be justified by the bedrock principles and sources of common Buddhist teachings.

The spiritual significance of Buddhism is twofold: First, it is an organized religion, with its own unique teachings and cultural nuances, as reflected most vividly in the traditions of various Asian countries.

We see the flowering of these traditions in images, prayers, rituals, disciplines, and even many ways of thinking, feeling, and living.

Second, the overwhelming significance—and indeed, the essence—of Buddhist teachings is universal. Buddhism transcends culture and religion. We don't need to be Buddhist to enjoy peace, openness, love, and wisdom. We can use common images, words, and feelings to heal ourselves, especially if we have faith in them and in our own inner resources. The path to healing our minds and to the liberation of enlightenment is open to Buddhist and non-Buddhist alike.

Over the centuries, numerous sages have chronicled the teachings of Buddhism. Some of those teachings are meant for everyone, and others are intended more specifically as esoteric trainings. In the following pages, I refer to both types of teachings and also frequently quote from the common (sutric) scriptures. My main purpose is to indicate the basis of the healing approach in the common teachings. Another purpose is to build appreciation, trust, and confidence in both the teachings and the teachers. It can be so inspiring to hear timeless wisdom quoted directly from its source.

MENTAL AND EMOTIONAL CONDITIONS AS THE BASIS FOR PHYSICAL HEALING

To heal physical problems, according to the ancient Tibetan medical texts, we must deal with their primary causes—mental and emotional afflictions.

The ancient texts view the physical body as composed of four elements—namely, earth, water, fire, and air—which have hot and cold temperatures. When the elements of our bodies are balanced, we are in our natural healthy state. When there is disharmony among the elements, disease occurs.

Tibetan medical texts, as in the *Ayurveda*, speak of bodily functions as driven by three vital "humors" (*Nyes Pa* or *'Du Ba*), which are both substantial and energetic. These are derived from the four (or five) great elements—earth, water, fire, air, and space. The three humors are air (*rLung*), bile (*mKhris Pa*), and phlegm (*Bad Kan*). A body that has normal or balanced humors (*rNam Par Ma Gyur Ba*) is what we call healthy. A body with abnormal or imbalanced humors (*rNam Par Gyur Pa*) is sick.

The imbalanced air humor is the disordered air element. Its temperature can be either hot or cold. The imbalanced bile humor is the disordered fire element with a hot temperature. Imbalanced phlegm is the disordered earth and water elements with a cold temperature.

The three imbalances of the humors are caused by the negative emotions of the mind. The imbalance of air is caused by desire, greed, craving, and attachment. The imbalance of bile is caused by dislike, resentment, anger, hatred, and aggression. The imbalance of phlegm is caused by delusion, ignorance, and confusion.

The root of the negative emotions is grasping at "self." When we see a mental object as if it were a truly existing entity, we are grasping at it. As our minds tighten the grip of this grasping at "self," we suffer. The *Shedgyud*, one of the four preeminent medical texts of Tibet, says:

> *Not knowing of "the nonexistence of self"*
> *Is the "general cause" of all the illnesses. . . .*
> *The "specific causes" of the illnesses are*
> *Aggression, greed, and confusion, which are caused by ignorance [of "no self"].*
> *They [in turn] produce the humors of air, bile, and phlegm.*
> *The "direct sources" of illness are the air, bile, and phlegm humors:*
> *Since the balanced humors are the basis of illnesses,*
> *The imbalanced humors are the very illnesses*
> *As they torment and endanger the body and life.*
> *[a] Imbalanced bile burns the energy of the body.*
> *It is accompanied by heat, the quality of the fire element.*
> *It is centered in the lower body but inflames the upper body.*
> *All the heat-related sicknesses come from this.*
> *[b] Imbalanced phlegm diminishes the heat of the body.*
> *It is heavy and cool, the qualities of the earth and water elements.*
> *It centers in the upper body but descends to the lower body.*
> *Cold-related sicknesses come from none but this.*
> *[c] Imbalanced air generates either heat or cold;*
> *It would assist the sun [energy] to burn and the moon to cool.*
> *It pervades the whole body: upper and lower, externally and internally.*
> *It stirs up either heat or cold, causing all the sicknesses.*[1]

HEALING AS A TRADITIONAL
BUDDHIST TEACHING

The cornerstone of Buddhism is the four noble truths: the truth of suffering, the recognition of its causes, the knowledge that suffering can be ended, and the end of suffering through the liberation of awakening.

I have spoken often in this book about the need to release the grasping qualities of our minds and about how letting go of grasping at "self" is the best way to heal suffering.

The traditional teachings speak in terms of the letting go that can ultimately result in total liberation as a form of healing. The process is comparable to a physician's healing sickness. The more we can release grasping, the "healthier" we will be. Asanga, who founded the Mind Only school of Buddhism, says it like this:

> As it is necessary to diagnose the sickness, to abandon its cause,
> Attain the happiness of good health, and apply medicine for it,
> The suffering should be recognized, the cause should be abandoned,
> The remedy for cessation should be applied, and cessation attained.[2]

THE ANCIENT ORIGINS OF
GUIDED MEDITATION

It is sometimes mistakenly thought that the practice of guided meditation is a recent development or that it was perhaps invented as a so-called New Age approach to contemplation. But guided meditation has long been an important part of Buddhist tradition, in Tibet and elsewhere.

In particular, chanting can be considered very much a guided meditation. Chants are prayers to Buddhas or aspirations for the good of all, and the act of saying these prayers out loud increases the power of the meditation. In addition, most chants are intended to instruct or guide ourselves or others on a meditative path, step by step.

According to the Venerable Thich Nhat Hanh, Buddhists used guided meditation even in the time of the Buddha:

> The sutra for Sickness and Dying . . . records the guided medita-
> tion that Sariputra used to help the layman Anathapindika when

Appendix 1

he was lying on his sickbed. The Venerable Sariputra guided Anathapindika step by step until he [Anathapindika] was able to transform his fear of death.[3]

COMBINING TEACHINGS FROM MANY SOURCES INTO ONE MEDITATIVE TRAINING

The twelve stages of healing meditation in this book don't come from one particular Buddhist text or teaching but from many different sources. I simply compiled and arranged these teachings as steps along one path of healing meditation.

There is plenty of precedent for this in Buddhism. For instance, when Atisha (982–1055), the great Indian Buddhist master, arrived in Tibet in 1042, he was impressed with the vast knowledge of the Tibetan scholar Rinchen Zangpo (958–1051). Atisha remarked, "What's the point of an old man like me coming to Tibet and enduring so much hardship, since it already has great scholars like you?" And Atisha asked, "How do you put all these teachings into practice?" Rinchen Zangpo answered, "We practice each teaching separately as [the texts] teach." Atisha retorted, "You are wrong. Now I know why I had to come." Then he wrote his famous text *Bodhipathapradipa* (The Lamp of the Path of Enlightenment) and put all the Buddha's teachings into a single path of training.

THE TEACHINGS OF COMMON (SUTRA) AND ESOTERIC (TANTRA) BUDDHISM

As a devotee of esoteric training, I want to give you a glimpse of the teachings that inspired me to write about healing and then indicate how their overall approach is reflected in the common teachings.

The esoteric teachings that are related to healing include the Vajrasattva (Buddha of Purification) meditation on purification and on receiving the four empowerments, which are the blessings of body, speech, mind, and wisdom.

In the esoteric teachings (Tantra):

• You view all as one in having enlightened nature, the utmost peace, joy, and omniscience.

183

- You receive blessings in the form of light, nectar, fire, or wind and purify or dispel the impurities of your body and mind and the world.
- You receive the blessings of the four sacred aspects of the Buddha or an enlightened sage: the changeless vajra body; the ceaseless vajra speech; the vajra mind, which is the union of bliss and openness; and the primordially pure vajra wisdom.
- You use the energy of blissful heat of the body as the means of awakening the union of blissful and open wisdom of your body and mind.
- You meditate on awakening various aspects of your body, mind, and phenomenal objects as the various forms and qualities of the Buddha and pure land.
- You transform the energies of both positive and negative, love and anger, and wrath and peace as the means of realizing the absolute nature, ultimate joyful peace.
- You meditate on seeing the body and matter as the indestructible buddha body of light, the union of appearances and openness. You hear speech and air or energy as the powerful buddha speech, the union of sound and openness. You experience mind and thought as omniscient buddha wisdom, the union of great bliss and openness.
- You attain enlightenment through the esoteric meditations on energy (*rLung*), bliss (*bDe Ba*), and heat (*gTum Mo*). Such meditations heal not only mental and emotional afflictions but physical ones, too. Padma Karpo writes, "By maintaining heat [with bliss] and maturing the energies, no afflictions, such as sickness and old age, will be able to harm you."[4]

  The energy of heat and bliss is developed through the discipline of the mind. Situ Tenpe Nyinched writes, "If you have mastery over your mind, you will have power over your energy. Then heat will develop and bliss will arise in you."[5]
- You remain in awareness of the union of all things as one, the universal truth, without conceptualizing things in terms of subject-object duality.

In order to practice esoteric teachings such as those just outlined, you must begin by being initiated into the path. If the initiation is properly performed—and I emphasize that it must be properly done—the innate wisdom of your mind will be awakened. Typically this will

184

be only a flash of the experience of your mind's true wisdom nature. Then you must perfect that awakening by meditation, using the very awakened wisdom as the cause, basis, and means of training.

In the common teachings (sutra), you train in generating a positive attitude and a loving and devotional heart. You dedicate your life to beneficial and compassionate activities in order to awaken your wisdom mind. You are undertaking such training not for yourself but for the sake of bringing peace and joy to all beings.

Many of the meditations in esoteric and common teachings are similar in form or structure. The differences lie in their depth, scope, and power. In esoteric training, a meditator uses the wisdom itself, which is awakened in the initiation and then perfected in meditation. In common training, a meditator employs the conceptual mind to bring about the realization of wisdom.

Most important, whereas the meditations in this book were inspired by esoteric teachings, I have presented here only the meditations that can also be found in the common teachings. These meditations employ the conceptual mind and feelings as the means of training, not the wisdom mind, which is beyond the range of most uninitiated meditators. The meditations in this book are open to all, initiated or uninitiated, and can benefit anyone who wants to perform them.

Esoteric meditators will find that these meditations have qualities similar to esoteric meditations. So even if you are advanced in your training, the healing meditations given here can be used as esoteric meditations, too.

SOURCES OF HEALING

The following is a sampling of the many nectarlike Buddhist sources on which the meditations in this book are based. The scriptural quotations are taken from common teachings.

THE VIEW THAT ALL PHENOMENA AND BEINGS ARE PURE AND HAVE BUDDHA NATURE AND BUDDHA QUALITIES

In the esoteric teachings of Buddhism, one recognizes the perfection of the buddha wisdom and buddha qualities of all things, as they truly are.

In the common teachings, the view is that every being possesses buddha nature and buddha qualities and should seek the means to awaken that true nature and those pure qualities. Asangha writes:

> *The [ultimate] body of the Buddha prevails [in all].*
> *The ultimate nature is [in all] without distinctions.*
> *All beings have the lineage [of becoming Buddha].*
> *Beings always possess buddha nature.*[6]

VISUALIZATION OF THE DIVINE PRESENCE

In esoteric training, visualization of all appearances as the divine presence is one of the important meditations for purifying our own negative perceptions and transforming them into pure qualities, as they are.

In common teachings, too, we find trainings on seeing or visualizing the world as infinite Buddha manifestations. A sutra says:

> *I think that on each atom, there are as many Buddhas as the number of*
> *   atoms of the world,*
> *Sitting in the midst of [an ocean of] children [disciples].*
> *Likewise, the entire sphere*
> *Is filled with [an infinite cloud of] Buddhas. . . .*
> *On each atom, there are as many pure lands as the number of atoms of*
> *   the worlds.*
> *In each pure land, there are infinite Buddhas*
> *Sitting in the midst of the children [disciples] of the Buddhas.*
> *May I see them and perform the enlightened activities with them.*[7]

SEEING YOUR OWN BODY AS A PURE BODY

The important aspects of esoteric training are: seeing your body as a divine body of light, sending and receiving blessing lights as the means of purifying defilements, healing sickness, and achieving the attainments.

Receiving blessings in the form of light or nectar from a blessed source and sending blessings to others are taught in common teachings, too. A sutra says:

> *Projecting immeasurable colorful lights [from the body of the Buddha,]*
> *Wishes of the beings were fulfilled, as they wished.*[8]

186

A sutra says:

The lights [of the Buddha], even if no Buddha is present,
Manifesting as the pure body of the Buddha,
Reveal the most profound teachings.[9]

A sutra says:

From every pore of Buddha's body,
Projecting hundreds of thousands of rays of light,
[He] cleared [gSal] all.[10]

A sutra says:

Great lights [came from the Buddha and] filled [the ten directions].
Beings who saw the lights and were touched by them were assured
of attaining the unexcelled full enlightenment.[11]

A sutra says:

Contemplating in an absorption called the Play of the Lion, the
Buddha displayed miracles. . . . The earth shook in six kinds of
waves. . . . [As the result of buddha lights and miracles,] people
who were sick were healed. . . . Beings experienced such total bliss-
fulness as an ascetic experiencing the bliss of an absorption.[12]

Great Master Shantarakshita writes:

To the King of the Healers [the Healing Buddha],
Who liberates beings through the light of his body, I pay homage.[13]

I have mentioned in this book that in their true quality, the five
elements are five colored lights. This view is based on an esoteric text
of Tibetan Buddhism. In *Serthreng*, it is said:

Due to grasping at the "self" of blue, white,
Yellow, red, and green lights,
They have spontaneously appeared as the five gross elements—
Namely, space, water, earth, fire, and air.[14]

I couldn't find any source in the common teachings that expounds the same view. However, even modern physics seems more or less in agreement that matter is another form of energy (or light). So I hope that bringing this view of light to the attention of readers is not a breach of the discipline of esoteric teachings, since matter being a form of light is now common knowledge.

Heat or Warmth

Generating extraordinary heat and energy through esoteric exercises of the vajra body is a special skill in esoteric trainings. But generating healthy heat (fire) that travels with the breathing (air) and is led by awareness of the mind is simply the way that the body stays alive and healthy. We will die not only if breathing stops but if heat ceases. So using heat is not only spiritual but is also a common way of healing. Khenpo Ngakchung writes, "According to Abhidharma[kosha], life is the duration of the coexistence of heat and consciousness."[15]

Bliss or Joy

The supreme union of emptiness and "great bliss" or great joy through the power of the chakras, channels, and energy of the vajra body is one of the essential esoteric trainings.

Likewise, in many common teachings, bliss is presented as the buddha blessings that we receive, but its caliber and the way that it is generated differ from the bliss energy derived from the esoteric meditations. A sutra says, "The light [of the Infinite Light Buddha] is immaculate and generates bliss in the bodies and joy in the minds [of whomever it has touched]."[16]

Jey Tsongkhapa writes, "The light of [the Infinite Light Buddha] is unstained like a crystal ball, expansive [as the] sky; it creates bliss in the body, joy in the mind, and great joy in whomever it touches."[17]

Again, Jey Tsongkhapa writes, "When the body and mind become proficient [in absorption] and joyful bliss is experienced, the absorption becomes tranquillity."[18]

Air or Breathing

Using the breath as waves, the means of refining and perfecting mental and physical energies, is one of the important meditations in esoteric

188

practice to melt the mind and air into the great blissful primordial wisdom.

Breathing is essential to life and can also be considered a common form of healing. Breathing is one of the functions that most intimately draws together mind and body. Our breath carries waves of air and warmth that enliven our blood and keep it circulating. Thus, using the breath to refine and channel heat and bliss energies is a commonsense and universal approach to healing.

LIGHT OR NECTAR AS THE MEANS OF BLESSING

Both esoteric and common teachings share the practice of seeing and receiving blessings of the Buddhas in the form of light or nectar to heal pain and confusion and attain spiritual accomplishments. The following quotations are from common sources.

Karma Chakme writes:

Meditate that lapis-colored light comes from [the Healing Buddha],
Enters into the bodies of oneself and those who are seeking healing, and
That all the diseases are evaporated like frost at the touch of sunlight.[19]

Chogyur Lingpa writes:

The stream of nectar descends from the body of Tara, entering through the crown of the head of myself and those who are seeking healing, fills our bodies with it, and transmits all the blessings to us.[20]

Mipham Rinpoche writes:

Think that the great rays of colorful wisdom light from the body of the Buddha [have come and have entered into you and all beings]. [By the touch of the wisdom light,] all the defilements of yourself and of all beings are purified, and the virtues of the path of Mahayana are perfected.[21]

The third Dodrupchen writes:

Praying with one-pointed mind, [think that] the mind streams of the Buddhas are invoked. From their bodies, rays of light have come [and have entered into us]. All the sufferings of oneself and other beings are pacified, and all our wishes are fulfilled.[22]

THE SOUND OF AH

According to esoteric teachings, AH is the syllable that represents the speech of the Buddhas. It is the sound of openness (emptiness) that is uncreated and unceasing. It is also the source of all sounds and words, just as space is necessary for all material objects to exist. A tantra says:

> *AH is the supreme of all the syllables.*
> *It is the meaningful and sacred syllable.*
> *It doesn't produce or give birth to anything.*
> *It doesn't convey any designations.*
> *[But] it is the supreme source of all expressions.*[23]

According to common teaching, AH is unborn and is the source of all expressions, just as space is the source for all forms. A sutra says, "AH is the door of all, as it is unborn."[24]

The sound AH is the essence of all the teachings on Perfect Wisdom (prajnaparamita). The longest version of the *Perfect Wisdom Sutras* is *Shatasahasrika*, in twelve volumes. A sutra says:

> The Buddha said, "For the benefit of beings, remember that the single syllable is the Mother, the Perfect Wisdom. That is the AH. . . ."
> Bodhisattvas [who were present] realized the meaning of the Perfect Wisdom, and all rejoiced at the teaching.[25]

TEACHINGS ON THE HEALING BUDDHA

Tibetan scholars place the three canonical liturgies[26] on the Healing Buddha in the esoteric (*rgyud*) section of Kanjur. The Healing Buddha liturgy by master Shantarakshita[27] is placed among the esoteric teachings of Tenjur. However, according to the fifth Dalai Lama,[28] Shantarakshita's liturgy is mainly a common teaching, so it could belong to both common and esoteric teachings.

MANTRA AND DHARANI

Most of the mantras and name-prayers (Skt. *dharani*, Tib. *mTshan gzungs*) belong to the lore of esoteric teachings. These mystic syllables, words, and sounds are in Sanskrit or in one of the mystical languages. In essence, they are the wisdom heart energies of the deities and the channels of the mystical blessings.

Some mantras and many name-prayers are in Tibetan Buddhist common teachings, too. These Sanskrit name-prayers invoke the blessings of the Buddhas. They are the sound of peace, joy, and power. Sometimes you will find the same name-prayer in both esoteric and common teachings, but they are used for different ways of practice.

ONENESS

The realization and awareness of oneness, in which subject-object duality and discriminations do not exist, is the highest esoteric training.

In common teachings, too, the meditations on the oneness of the mind (subject) and the object or action are among the most important trainings. A sutra says, "When the practitioner breathes in or out with the awareness of joy or happiness, . . . at that time he abides peacefully in the observation of the feeling in the feeling."[29]

Explaining these lines of the *Anapanasati-sutra*, Thich Nhat Hanh writes, " 'observing the feelings in feelings' . . . is that the subject of the observation and the object of the observation are not [to] be regarded as two separate things. . . . Non-duality is the key word."[30]

INTERDEPENDENCE OF THE MEANS OF HEALING

For healing, it is most effective to activate all the related components of the body and mind, in meditation as well as in the activities of daily life. Different means of healing should be called into action to function as a team. The reason for this is that nothing functions independently; rather, things function through interdependent causation. Nagarjuna writes:

There is nothing
That doesn't [arise or function] through dependent causation.[31]

THE ACCESSIBILITY OF COMMON BUDDHIST MEDITATIONS TO ALL WHO ARE OPEN

Common (or sutric) Buddhist teachings are open to all whose minds are open to them.

It is also true that becoming a Buddhist can be a great support on the path to liberation. Traditionally, we become Buddhists by taking the precepts of "going for refuge" in a ceremony. This is how we make a commitment to the Buddha as our teacher, to Buddhism as the path of our spiritual journey, and to other Buddhists as our community.

Becoming Buddhists establishes us as part of a living spiritual tradition and is a powerful exercise that inspires our minds and launches us on a positive life's journey.

Such faith is not a way of submitting ourselves to someone else, an external entity, but rather an important means of establishing confidence, a refuge, in ourselves.

If we could develop the habit of liking the teachings and wanting their benefits, and if we could cultivate a mind that trusts in such a path, we would start to loosen our mental grasping at a "self." Then our negative emotions would ease, and awareness of wisdom would shine forth in us.

However, it is also quite true that everyone has buddha nature, even those who are not interested in Buddhism or have never even heard of it. The enlightened nature is the birthright of all.

What matters is mental attitude, not necessarily ceremonies or even the religion to which we belong. With the right attitude, whatever path we choose will lead us to the result that we wish. A sutra says:

> [Attainment of] the truth depends on the conditions.
> It depends on [the conditions of] mental attitude.
> [So] whatever aspiration you make
> Will bring the results you have wished for.[32]

Of course, religious devotion can be a great help. If our minds are open to the Buddha, and if we are thinking about him, the Buddha is present before us, for the Buddha is not someone outside ourselves but rather a reflection of our true nature. A sutra says:

> Whoever thinks of the Buddha,
> The Buddha is present in front of him or her.
> He grants his blessings and
> Dispels all flaws.[33]

If our hearts are filled with genuine caring for others with love and compassion, at that very moment we have become not only Buddhists but bodhisattvas. Shantideva writes:

When the mind of enlightenment is born in us, at that very moment,
We who are disheartened by confinement in the prison of samsara
Will become known as the heirs of the Buddhas
And be honored by the world of men and gods.[34]

So if we have opened our minds with the thoughts of liking, wanting, and trusting in the path and goal of healing meditation, we are already followers of the enlightened path, or Buddhism. Whoever does this is a Buddhist, regardless of whether he or she has taken that designation.

On the other hand, even if we designate ourselves as Buddhists, we can hardly claim to be true Buddhists if we ignore the right path and instead grasp after money, power, pleasures, and ideas.

There have been many enlightened people from other traditions and religions. Tibetan Buddhists are impressed when they hear of anyone who has led a saintly life or displayed miraculous or holy powers or simply manifested great joy or peace in his or her actions or very way of being. A Tibetan would typically say, "He or she must be a manifestation of the Buddhas," or "It must be the blessings of the Buddhas." Underneath these simple, pious sentiments is a profound and encompassing understanding of spirituality. For Buddhism is universal in nature: the Buddha and buddha blessings are open to all, no matter their religious designation.

THE ELEMENTS OF NATURE AS THE MEANS OF HEALING

Mahayana Buddhists believe that the whole universe is pure and perfect in its true nature and true quality. The problem is not in the phenomena of the world and what they are or are not but rather in how your mind perceives them. If you see the world around you as a source of peace and joy, it will become a blessing and benefit for you. If your mind is pure and open, a healing object could be a Buddhist image or a tree. The Buddha said:

193

For those whose minds are pure, even if they live in a world different from the Buddha's, he will appear before them. . . . For them, the treasures of dharma are present in mountains, the foot of mountains, and in trees.[35]

The great master Shantideva makes the following aspiration:

May all embodied beings hear
The sound of dharma without cessation
From the birds and the trees
And from lights and the sky.[36]

Many nonreligious people cannot tolerate healing methods with religious overtones, even if those methods are beneficial. Many religious people cannot tolerate nonreligious healing methods, even if they are beneficial. If either of these descriptions fits you, you need to work on letting go of your attitudes of insecurity and self-protection.

Everyday objects and the elements of nature can be important means of healing the suffering of beings. This beautiful passage from Shantideva expresses the aspiration of a bodhisattva who wishes to become the source of healing for beings:

As long as there are people who are sick,
And until they are healed,
May I become the doctors and the medicines.
And may I become the nurses for them. . . .
May I become the protectors for all the defenseless beings,
The guides for all the travelers,
The ships, boats, and bridges
For all who wish to cross [oceans and rivers],
The lands for those who seek lands [on which to disembark],
The lamps for those who [are in darkness and] desire light,
The houses and mattresses [for the tired],
The servants for all [the old and sick] who are in need of care,
Wish-fulfilling precious jewels and excellent vessels,
Ascetic powers and medicines [for healing the sick],
Wish-fulfilling trees,
Wish-fulfilling cows,
The great elements such as earth [water, fire, air]

As well as the space [that supports the existence of all beings].
May I always be the source for sustaining
All the infinite beings.[37]

Dharma is not just words in scripture or a book but the knowledge and experience of those words and their meaning. Dharma is not just the attainment of some spiritual feats but the ultimate healing of peace and wisdom.

If your speech is proper, spoken properly for the proper purpose, it is right speech, and it is a Buddhist training. If you see, think, feel, and believe in the right way, you are on the path of enlightenment, or Buddhism, even if you don't call it by that name.

So if you could see any object whatever—and especially a positive object—as the source of peace and joy, then it becomes a source of peace. If you see things negatively, even if an image of the Buddha were before you, it would bring hardly any benefit.

HEALING THE MIND AS THE WAY TO HEAL OUR PROBLEMS

We can't solve or heal all our problems by dealing with them individually, because they are numerous. Healing our own minds is the right approach to negative circumstances. Shantideva says:

The sources of foes [problems] are as unlimited as space;
They cannot possibly all be overcome.
Yet if you just overcome the thought of disliking,
That will be equal to overcoming all the sources of problems.

[For example,] where is the leather
With which one can cover the earth?
But wearing a leather sandal
Is equal to covering the whole earth with leather.[38]

CULTIVATING A PEACEFUL MIND

It is so important to transform our habitual negative habits into positive habits; otherwise, we have little chance of achieving peace in our lives. If our minds are filled with negative concepts, we are building a prison of self-limiting attitudes. Shantideva was clear about the dangers of allowing negative emotions to take hold of our lives:

> *If I harbor the painful thoughts of hatred,*
> *I will never experience peace, and*
> *I will have no [mental] joy or [physical] pleasure.*
> *Even sleep and strength will be absent from my life.*[39]

Such common teachings warn us about grasping at negative emotions and attitudes, but how can we experience true peace? Sometimes we seem to glimpse our peaceful minds, but then the experience slips away. One reason for this is the tendency to grasp not just at the negative but at the positive, too. If we experience joy, we try to hold on to it or greedily want more of it. Or we mistake excitement and fascination for peace and grasp at that. Or we are upset by something we don't like that spoils our peace of mind and refuse to work with that circumstance to make the best of it. Then the wheel of craving and avoiding starts to turn.

It is better to cultivate peace, even if we tend to grasp at it, than to stay imprisoned by negative attitudes and emotions. If we practice the experience of peace in our minds, then gradually we can learn to loosen our grasping attitudes. If we can deepen our experience of peace, gradually our lives will be transformed. The key is to cultivate a peaceful mind. This is the way to be happier. It is also the way to liberation. The Buddha said:

> *One whose mind is enjoying peace*
> *Enters the state of ultimate peace and joy.*[40]

TURNING ANY POSITIVE ACTIVITY INTO A BUDDHIST DISCIPLINE

Any action or activity, if it is positive or at least neutral, could be considered a Buddhist meditation on healing. The Buddhist practices of positive perception and mindfulness are the foundations for transforming daily life into a healing path.

Negative actions harm ourselves or others. Neutral actions are neither harmful nor beneficial to ourselves or others. Positive actions benefit ourselves or others. For centuries, Buddhists have used positive action in their everyday activities as a practice on the path to peace and wisdom.

There are so many positive practices that are applicable to every aspect of living, from getting up in the morning to working, walking, playing, reading, and falling asleep at night. Rather than quote any sources or sage advice, I am simply going to enumerate some of the common practices for just one activity—eating. Eating is common to all beings—to humans, animals, and insects alike. It is a blessing to eat food and even more of a blessing to enjoy our food with awareness and appreciation, no matter how rich or humble our food may be. Eating also is necessary to sustain the health of our bodies, which is one of the main themes of this book.

Here are some of the Buddhist practices on eating:

- By eating food with mindfulness, we can cultivate awareness, calmness, peace, and joy.
- By eating food with thankfulness to all who made a contribution to bringing this great gift to our tables, we can cultivate the quality of love and appreciation of others.
- By eating food with the wish to sustain our bodies as vessels for serving many, we can cultivate a vision beyond our restricted self-concerns and a habit of dedicating mind and body to a greater goal.
- By eating food with gratitude as a gift to our own bodies, which are vessels for such an amazing life, we cultivate a tendency to feel friendship, appreciation, and respect for our own bodies rather than grasping, craving, or hatred.
- By eating food with the intention of nourishing the bacteria that live in our bodies, we cultivate a sense of purpose, love, and generosity.
- By eating food with the attitude of offering it to the divine body or to the divinity in our bodies, as many meditators do, we cultivate great merits and blessing energies.
- By eating food with right thinking and feeling, we transform ourselves into persons of peace and joy. These qualities benefit us and could transform us into sources of peace and joy for many others.

Appendix 2

ANSWERS TO SOME FREQUENTLY ASKED QUESTIONS

A FTER *The Healing Power of Mind* was published, I enjoyed receiving letters from readers and meeting many people at workshops. The reaction to the first book inspired me in my work on this sequel. In the new book, I wanted to elaborate on the healing meditations, discuss some new subjects, and also answer some questions about healing.

It is so gratifying to hear firsthand that the healing methods have been helpful. At the workshops, many people unfamiliar with the healing meditations appeared to get some immediate benefit. For example, some people gave themselves so fully to the visualizations that they strongly felt they were actually entering into the boundless cells of light with the feeling of awe, openness, and joy. It's this kind of wholehearted involvement with the meditations that reaps great rewards, especially when the practice is kept up consistently.

Among the inspiring things I heard from readers were: "Your book helped me when I was going through such difficult times." "Your book helped me to learn how appealing Buddhism is. It is all about improving every step of our own everyday life, enjoying the life that we have, and making the best of it." "Your book has been a constant support and inspiration on my journey out of deep depression." "My mother has never been open to any religion and never to Buddhism. But she is enjoying your book." "Your book was very helpful for my mother and all of us while our mother was sick and after her death." And most amazingly, someone came up after a workshop and said, "I have come to see you because your book saved my life."

A Catholic gentleman wrote that until he heard me interviewed on the radio and read my book, he "never took to heart the key to salvation that is revealed by all the world's major religions: selflessness. . . . [A]t least now I am paying attention to this most critical aspect of our existence." Although the book is based on Buddhist principles, it inspired him to pay more attention to his own faith. I found his reaction very gratifying, since it indicates that the book's approach is universal and relevant to all who are open, not just Buddhists.

Then there was the couple with experience in a twelve-step treatment program for addiction. They were very interested in the Buddhist use of a "source of power" and other external sources for healing. This is similar to the twelve-step program, which advises its participants to rely on a "higher power" for help but leaves it up to individuals to interpret spirituality in whatever way they see fit. Regardless of whether someone believes in God, the support of an external source can be extremely helpful. In Buddhism, the power of mind is the ultimate source of our strength and wisdom. Even so, most of us need some positive source outside ourselves to encourage our inner resources.

I was also struck by the strong faith that some workshop participants had in prayer. They sent healing waves to their friends during the guided meditations. Later they found out that these friends had felt a sense of well-being at that particular time, even though they had no idea that anybody was sending healing blessings to them. Typically, the main benefit of meditation is for the meditator. But if people have faith in the power of prayer for others, and if they want to share the benefits of meditation with others, this can inspire them in their meditation.

The following are my answers to some of the memorable questions people have asked about the healing meditations.

Why do you focus more on receiving healing blessings yourself than on giving them to others?

When we try to begin our journey on a spiritual path, finding excuses not to move forward is a typical trap for many of us. When we

200

are not pursuing any spiritual path, we don't even think that much about caring for others, but when we are at the starting point of some worthwhile journey, we immediately begin hearing, "Oh, you're so selfish. You're enjoying peace and joy, while many others are suffering. That's not fair!" That freezes us where we are and prevents us from making any progress. At this point, we have to remember two things:

1. In order to help or heal others, we must first gain the benefit of healing blessings ourselves. It is like wanting to give money to a needy person: first, we must have or make some money, because only then can we give it away.
2. Yes, according to Buddhism, especially Mahayana Buddhism, the best spiritual training is to serve the needs of others, the mother beings, with no selfish motivations. That means that our purpose in generating peace and joy in ourselves must be for the sake of others, or at least that must be our aim.

Thus, we must create and feel peace and joy in ourselves with no hesitation. When we have gained these benefits, we must share them with others, with the greatest joy.

Also, we must understand that if we can generate peace and joy in ourselves even for our own sake, we will have an enjoyable life. If we have peace, spontaneously all our words and actions will be expressions of peace and joy. Then, even if we are not actively sharing peace or trying to help others, our good qualities will still have a positive effect on many around us.

So it is important to be impatient with ourselves when we are indulging in evil thoughts and deeds. However, we must be patient with ourselves when we are about to swim into peace and joy.

Why do you rely on conceptual healing instead of the meditation on the non-dual state that transcends everything?

If we have meditative experience of nonduality, free from concepts, then we must use that experience to heal problems, as nondual meditation is the most powerful means of healing. But merely having conceptual ideas of nonduality or the ambition to do such meditation will not equip us to transcend everything or share the benefits of higher meditation with others.

This book is not for highly accomplished meditators, for whom these exercises may not be of much use. This book is for the majority of people like us, for we perceive mental objects dualistically and emotionally crave or dislike them. We need to allow ourselves to proceed step by step from where we are.

First, we need to heal negative thoughts, emotions, and feelings with positive thoughts and feelings. When our thoughts and feelings are more positive, then and only then are we ready to go beyond the positive by realizing and dwelling in an open, nondual state.

Otherwise, by merely entertaining the idea of doing only high meditations, we may avoid pursuing any meditations at all, even simpler ones, and end up by doing nothing in our lives. If we can't afford bread, how can we live on cake?

Are there many different methods of healing in Tibetan Buddhism?

There are thousands of different methods of healing in Tibetan Buddhism. A wide variety of trainings is used to generate and strengthen healing, such as visualizing peaceful or wrathful images; saying various prayers, name-prayers, syllables, and sounds; and performing different physical rituals and mental exercises.

In Tibet, I witnessed many simple people who repeated their prayers millions of times, even though they had no philosophical understanding of meditation. But they had such strong faith in the power of prayer that they could heal all kinds of sicknesses. Mystical objects, deity images, and mystical diagrams blessed by powerful masters were used to prevent and heal many misfortunes.

There are so many ways of generating devotional trust and so many sources and means of healing. We could receive healing blessings in the forms of light, water, air, earth, sound, and feeling. We could develop faith in divine presences or an accomplished master in visualized form or in person.

The means and methods of healing are not lacking. What's lacking is our understanding and dedication and our faith in the power of healing.

Do you need permission to share the healing power with others?

According to Buddhism, there is no need to get permission from others to offer anything beneficial to them. However, if you feel that you must have permission, then it might be better to get it. Otherwise, the mental block of your doubting mind could hinder your sharing the benefits of healing.

I must add that if anyone really cares that much about the need for permission to share something good, then it would really be a better idea to get permission before you send someone such negative energies as your anger, attachment, jealousy, and ego! So ask the target of your energy, "May I get angry with you?" before experiencing such an emotion.

Do we need to be careful about what wishes we make?

Wishing harm to someone could cause that person harm, especially if he or she is open and vulnerable. But if you are harboring a selfish attitude when you make such a wish, then greater harm will come to you than to anybody else.

Although some call it negative prayer, *prayer* is the wrong word for it, since prayers are always for good. Making negative wishes and expressing them in words is a curse, not a prayer.

Making any good wish is always positive, even if it is hard to accomplish. Among the traditional Buddhist wishes are: "Until every being has attained buddhahood, may I live in the suffering world for the sake of all the mother beings"; "May I give all the merits that I have to all"; "May I take all the pain and causes of pain of others to myself." Such wishes, instead of causing negative effects, will cause great progress in your spiritual journey.

However, if you harbor doubt and hesitation, and fear that such a wish might cause a negative reaction in you, then that could have an ill effect, not because of the wish itself but because of your mental doubts.

I don't want to rely on any person or thing outside myself. How can I appreciate external sources as pure?

In truth, if you can't appreciate positive external sources, you won't be able to appreciate your own positive inner qualities, either. At the moment, you may have little capacity for appreciation. Appreciation is a mental quality that you can develop, and it is very helpful to do so. If you have it, then you can appreciate everyone and everything according to its qualities. This does not make you dependent on others or the product of anything external.

NOTES

In the following notes, the titles of works cited are indicated by abbreviations, the key to which can be found in the Bibliography. For example, "KL" stands for *sKyid sDug Lam 'Khyer Gyi Man Ngag*. When a work in traditional Tibetan pagination is cited, the title abbreviation is followed by the folio number and the letter *a* or *b*, depending on whether the referenced material is on the front or back of the folio. This is followed by the line number (for example, KL, 1b/2).

When an English language source is cited, the title abbreviation is followed by the page number (for example, WPT, 173).

NOTES FOR INTRODUCTION

1. WPT, 173.
2. KL, 1b/2.

NOTES FOR CHAPTER 1

1. CT, 244a/1.
2. KL, 5a/2.
3. BC, 32b/1.
4. BC, 97b/2.
5. CT, 219b/6.
6. EI, 177.
7. Introduction to HPM, xi.

8. DT, 200a/7.
9. DT, 199a/1.
10. IO, 12.
11. NP, 609.
12. KL, 2b/4.
13. KL, 1a/5.
14. MSM, 68.
15. KL, 3b/5.

Note for Chapter 2

1. BC, 46b/5.

Note for Chapter 4

1. I have paraphrased Dr. Radhakrishnan's remarks, based on my memory.

Note for Chapter 5

1. IC, 67.

Note for Chapter 6

1. MR, 47.

Notes for Chapter 8

1. CT, 219b/7.
2. KZK, 189a/6.
3. KZ, 262b/3.
4. Dr. D. T. Suzuki translates it as "Primal Vow" or "Primal Will." See BIL, 26.
5. DDM, 261b/1–263a/4.
6. The literal meaning of the name-prayer is as follows:

tadyatha:	Thus,
om (a + o + m = om)	speech, body, and mind of Buddha (or "O")

bhaishajye	of Healing
bhaishajye	of Healing
mahabhaishajye	of Great Healing,
raja	the King,
samudgate	the Fully Exalted
svaha	hail to (or "the pure word of truth"—a benediction)

Regarding "Thus": Tibetan: dPer na a'm 'di lta ste.

Regarding "of Healing": Grammatically, it is locative case: "in healing." In SBS, 679, *Bhaishajyeraja* is translated into Tibetan as "sman gyi rgyal po" ("the King of Healing").

Regarding "the Fully Exalted": PK, 2b/3, says, "Byang ch'ub sems dpa' sman gyi rgyal po dang Byang ch'ub sems dpa' sman yang dag 'phags."

7. DB, 21a/6.
8. JK, 279a/4.

NOTE FOR CHAPTER 9

1. For details, see MM; TBD; and EJ, 51–77.

NOTES FOR APPENDIX 1

1. SG, 11a/5.
2. GB, 16b/7.
3. BL, 9.
4. CZ, 7b/1.
5. GZ, 38b/6.
6. GB, 6a/3.
7. ZC, 359a/1 and 360a/6.
8. OK, 196b/1.
9. OK, 201a/3.
10. OK, 224a/6.
11. TG, vol. Ka 5b/3.
12. TG, vol. Ka 6b/2–10a/2.
13. GT, 238a/6.
14. *gSer Phreng-tantra*, quoted in TDD, 46b/3.
15. NGR, 53a/5.
16. OKK, 251a/7.
17. ST, 92b/3.
18. LC, 305b/5.

19. RZ, 68b/5.
20. TN, 6a/3.
21. BT, 5b/3.
22. ZN, 5b/3.
23. TJ, 3a/3.
24. TG, vol. Ga 194a/5.
25. YC, 147b/3.
26. DDM, MG, and DBO.
27. DM.
28. YB, 16b/3.
29. FAB, 9.
30. FAB, 31.
31. TS, 15a/6.
32. JZK, 279a/4.
33. Quoted in BT, 3a/5.
34. BC, 3b/2.
35. SD, 96b/1.
36. BC, 134b/4.
37. BC, 20a/3.
38. BC, 33a/5.
39. BC, 47b/1.
40. CT, 242a/1.

Notes

GLOSSARY

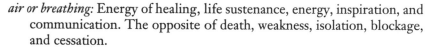

air or breathing: Energy of healing, life sustenance, energy, inspiration, and communication. The opposite of death, weakness, isolation, blockage, and cessation.

awareness: Mind of healing, being awake, alert, mindful, alive, and feeling. The opposite of unconsciousness, confusion, ignorance, sleepiness, spacing out, and distraction.

four healing powers: Positive images, words, feelings, and belief. These are the key to, and the heart of, the healing meditations presented in this book.

grasping at the positive: A useful alternative to grasping at the negative. If we have built habits of grasping at negative things and thoughts and can't function without being attached to them, it can be useful to grasp at positive things and thoughts. Positive sources will bring us some peace and strength, and then we may be able to work on releasing our grasping at positive things. It is helpful to use positive objects as stepping-stones for gradually releasing the grip of grasping.

grasping at self: The root of our mental ills, emotional afflictions, and physical sicknesses. It is the mind's tightness that comes from grasping at ourselves as "I," "my," and "me" and grasping at others as "this," "that," "he," "she," and so on. To the extent that the grip of grasping becomes tighter, our pain and confusion become more stressful and severe. To the extent that the grip of grasping is loosened, we will be healed and feel at ease. Total release of grasping is total liberation, the attainment of buddhahood.

healing energies: Qualities that can serve as the means of healing. In this book, the most important healing energies are heat and bliss. But the means of healing could also be the qualities of light, space, water, air, earth, and positive thoughts.

healing movements: Healing actions, the positive movements intrinsic to healing waves and change. Healing movements are associated with the acts of living, communicating, relating, progressing. The opposite of inflexibility, weakness, dullness, passivity, cessation, and death.

heat or warmth: Energy of healing, essential for life, digestive fire, health, force, and joy. The opposite of being cold, frozen, dead, sad, or sick.

joy or bliss: Energy of healing, positive energy, inspiration, force, and healing. The opposite of negativity, weakness, pain, sadness, dullness, and suffering.

oneness: Union with the result of meditation. At the end of each exercise, and also when all the stages of meditation are complete, we unite with the feeling of peace, joy, or whatever we are feeling, as water into water, and rest there for a while. This is how to sow the seed of meditation at a deeper level of the mind. However, an accomplished Buddhist meditator could spend the entire time of the meditation in the state of nonduality.

openness: Atmosphere or attitude of healing, awareness, peace, boundlessness. The opposite of restriction, tightness, closeness, limitation, bondage, bias, attachment, grasping, and egoism.

peace and joy: The goal of healing. Peace is being aware of peaceful experiences and expressions of our minds. It is not simply a neutral state of rest or the absence of thoughts or actions in a spaced-out, sleepy way, nor is it the mere absence of negative emotions and physical disharmonies. Joy is the awareness of freedom from conflict. There is no greater joy than the awareness of peace, which is boundless and open joy. When we are aware of peace, nothing can disturb us because of the strength that comes from this awareness.

positive object: Any object that causes peace and joy in us. Such an object is a true source of healing.

Furthermore, sources with spiritual significance and qualities will have a greater power of healing than ordinary positive images, if we believe in their power, because spiritual sources are born from deeper and more inward qualities and equipped with stronger power.

Spiritual sources could be actual objects or visualized images, sounds, feelings, holy places, blessed substances, spiritual people, prayers, spiritual beings, or meditation.

We use their power as the source and means of healing, as if the healing power came from them. Actually, the healing power comes from our own minds, and we are using external sources merely to support healing.

source of power: A positive presence. It can be a Buddha, a deity, an image, a prayer, an experience, or an idea. Or it could be a secular image, such as a beautiful flower, an open sky, a soothing sound, or a peaceful and joyful feeling. Any real or mental object will be a powerful source of healing if it has positive qualities and is appreciated by the mind as positive.

transformation: Converting our problems into positive experiences by the skillful use of images, words, feelings, and belief. For example, if we are facing pain, we can recall a peaceful or blissful experience from our past as the healing agent or focal point. Then we think and feel that the pain has soaked into this peaceful experience and melted and that the pain has become peaceful and blissful, like salt into water. The third Dodrupchen says this about transformation: "It is important to gain experience with a healing agent in advance. Then, with that healing agent, the transmutation of your problems will be highly effective" (KL, 3b/6).

BIBLIOGRAPHY

WORKS CITED WITH KEY TO ABBREVIATIONS

BC: *Byang Ch'ub Sems dPa'i sPyod Pa La 'Jug Pa* (Skt. *Bodhicharyavatara*), by Shantideva. Dodrupchen Monastery.

BIL: *Buddha of Infinite Light*, by Dr. D. T. Suzuki. Boston: Shambhala Publications, 1997.

BL: *The Blooming of a Lotus*, by Thich Nhat Hanh. Boston: Beacon Press, 1993.

BT: *Thub Ch'og Byin rLabs gTer mDzod*, by Mipham Jamyang Gyatso. Vol. 15, Jamgon Mipham Kabum. Dege edition.

CT: *Ch'ed Du brJod Pa'i Tshoms* (Skt. *Udanavarga*). Vol. Sa, mDo sDe, Kajur. Dege edition.

CZ: *Ch'os Drug bsDus Pa'i Zin Bris*, by Padma Karpo.

DB: *sMan Bla'i mDo Ch'og bsDus Pa bDud rTsi'i Bum bZang*, by Mipham Jamyang Gyatso. Vol. 27, Jamgon Mipham Kabum. Dege edition.

DBO: *De bZhin gShegs Pa'i Ting Nge 'Dzin Gyi sTobs bsKyed Pa Bai Durya'i Od Ches Bya Ba'i Zungs* (Skt. *Tathagata-vaiduryaprabha-nama-balad-hana-samadhi-dharani*). Vol. Da, rGyud 'Bum, Kajur. Dege edition.

DDM: *De bZhin gShegs Pa bDun Gyi sNgon Gyi sMon Lam Gyi Khyad Par rGyas Pa* (Skt. *Arya-saptatathagata-purvapranidhana-vishesavistara*). Vol. Da, rGyud 'Bum, Kajur. Dege edition.

DM: *De bZhin gShegs Pa bDun Gyi sNgon Gyi sMon Lam Gyi Khyad Par rGyas Pa'i mDo sDe'i Man Ngag* (Skt. *Saptatathagata-purvapranidhana-vishesavistara-sutrantopadesha*), by Bodhisattva (Shantarakshita). Vol. Pu, Gyud Drel, Kajur. Dege edition.

DT: *Dri Ma Med Pas bsTan Pa'i mDo* (Skt. *Vimalakirtinirdesha*). Vol. Ma, mDo sDe, Kajur. Dege edition.

EI: *Emotional Intelligence*, by Daniel Goleman. New York: Bantam, 1995.

EJ: *Enlightened Journey*, by Tulku Thondup. Boston: Shambhala Publications, 1995.

FAB: *The Sutra on the Full Awareness of Breathing* (Pali *Anapanasati-sutra*), translated with commentary by Thich Nhat Hanh. Berkeley, Calif.: Parallax Press, 1988.

GB: *Theg Pa Ch'en Po rGyud Bla Ma* (Skt. *Uttaratantra*), by Maitreyanatha. Vol. Phi, Sems Tsam, Tenjur. Dege edition.

GT: *De bZhin gShegs Pa brGyad La bsTod Pa* (Skt. *Ashtatathagata-stotra*), by Shantaraksita. Vol. Ka, bsTod Tshogs, Tenjur. Dege edition.

GZ: *Nges Don Phyag rGya Ch'en Po'i sMon Lam Gyi 'Grel Ba mCh'og Gi Zhal Lung*, by Situ Tenpe Nyinched.

HPM: *The Healing Power of Mind*, by Tulku Thondup. Boston: Shambhala Publications, 1996.

IC: *The Imitation of Christ*, by Thomas à Kempis. Notre Dame, Ind.: Ave Maria Press, 1996.

IO: *Ideas and Opinions*, by Albert Einstein. New York: Crown Trade Paperbacks, 1982.

JK: *'Jam dpal gyi sangs rgays kyi zhing gi yon tan dkod pa* (248b–297a). Vol. Ga, dKon brtsegs section, Kajur. Dege edition.

JZK: *'Jam dPal Gyi Sangs rGyas Kyi Zhing Gi Yon Tan bKod Pa* (Skt. *Manjushri-buddhaksetra-guna-vyuha*). Vol. Ga, dKon brTsegs, Kajur. Dege edition.

KL: *sKyid sDug Lam 'Khyer Gyi Man Ngag*, by Jigme Tenpe Nyima (the third Dodrupchen). Vol. Cha, rDro Grub Ch'en gSung 'Bum. Dodrupchen Rinpoche).

KZ: *sNying Thig sNgon 'Gro'i Khrid Yig Kun bZang Bla Ma'i Zhal Lung*, by Paltul Rinpoche. Sithron Mirig Petrun Khang, 1988.

KZK: *sNying Thig sNgon 'Gro'i Khrid Yig Kun bZang Bla Ma'i Zhal Lung Gi Khrid Yig*, by Pema Ledreltsal (Khenpo Ngagchung). Sithron Mirig Petrun Khang, 1992.

LC: *Byang Ch'ub Lam Rim Ch'e Ba*, by Jey Tsongkhapa. Vol. Pa, rJe'i gSung 'Bum.

MG: *bChom lDan 'Das sMan Gyi Bla Bai-durya Od Kyi rGyal Po'i sNgon Gyi sMon Lam Gyi Khyad Par rGyas Pa* (Skt. *Bhagavato-bhaisajyaguru-vaidurya-prabhasyapurva-pranidhana-vishesa-vistar a*). Vol. Da, rGyud 'Bum, Kajur. Dege edition.

MM: *The Mirror of Mindfulness: The Cycle of the Four Bardos*, by Tsele Natsok Rangtrol, translated by Erik Pema Kunsang. Boston: Shambhala Publications, 1989.

MR: *The Meaning of Relativity*, by Albert Einstein. Princeton, N.J.: Princeton University Press, 1972.

MSM: *Man's Search for Meaning*, by Viktor E. Frankl. New York: Washington Square Press, 1984.

NGR: *rTogs brJod Ngo mTshar sGyu Ma'i Rol Gar* (autobiography), by Pema Ledreltsal (Khenpo Ngagchung). Sonam Topgye.

NP: William Wordsworth, quoted in *The Norton Anthology of Poetry*. New York: Norton, 1975.

OK: *Od Zer Kun Du bKye Da bsTan Pa* (Skt. *Rashmisamantamukta-nirdesha*). Vol. Kha, dKon brTsegs, Kajur. Dege edition.

OKK: *Od dPag Med Kyi bKod Pa* (Skt. *Amitabhavyuha*). Vol. Ka, dKon brTsegs, Kajur. Dege edition.

PK: *Dam Pa'i Ch'os Padma dKar Po* (Skt. *Saddharmapundarika*). Vol. Ja, mDo sDe, Kajur. Dege edition.

RZ: *Ri Ch'os mTshams Kyi Zhal gDams*, by Karma Chagme (Trashi Jong).

SBS: *Sam Bod sKad gNyis Shan sByar* (Sanskrit Tibetan Dictionary). Kansu Mirig Petrun Khang, 1989.

SD: *bSod Nams Thams Chad bDus Pa'i Ting Nge 'Dzin* (Skt. *Sarvapunyasamuccayasamdhi*). Vol. Na, mDo sDe, Kajur. Dege edition.

SG: *bDud rTsi sNying Po Yan Lag brGyad Pa gSang Ba Man Ngag Gi rGyud Las Dum Bu gNyis Pa bShad Pa'i rGyud*, translated into Tibetan by Bairotsana and discovered as a Ter by Trawa Ngonshe (1012–1090?). Leh, India: Smanrtsis Shesrig Spendzod, 1978.

ST: *gSung Thor Bu*, by Jey Tsongkhapa. Vol. Kha, Jey Sungbum.

TBD: *The Tibetan Book of Living and Dying*, by Sogyal Rinpoche. San Francisco: HarperSanFrancisco, 1992.

TDD: *Tshig Don Rin Po Ch'e'i mDzod*, by Longchen Rabjam. Dodrupchen Rinpoche.

TG: *Shes Rab Kyi Pha Rol Du Phyin Pa sTong Phrag brGya Pa* (Skt. *Shatasahasrika-prajnaparamita*). Vol. Ka—Da and Ah, Sher Phyin, Kajur. Dege edition.

TJ: *'Jam dPal Gyi mTshan Yang Dag Par brJod Pa* (Skt. *Manjushrinamasamgiti*). Vol. Ka, rGyud, Kajur. Dege edition.

TN: *dGongs gTer sGrol Ma'i Zab Tig Las Mandala Ch'o Ga Tshogs gNyis sNying Po*, by Chogyur Lingpa.

TS: *dBu Ma rTsa Ba'i Tshig Leur Byas Pa Shes Rab* (Skt. *Prajna-nama-mula-madhyamaka-karika*), by Nagarjuna. Vol. Tsa, Uma, Tenjur. Dege edition.

WPT: *The Words of My Perfect Teacher*, by Paltul Rinpoche, translated by the Padmakara Translation Group. New York: HarperCollins, 1994.

YB: *bDe gShegs bDun Gyi mCh'od Pa'i Ch'og bsGrigs Yid bZhin dBang rGyal*, by Lobzang Gyatso (the fifth Dalai Lama), Sung Kama. Vol. Ka. Sonam T. Kazi.

YC: *Shes Rab Kyi Pha Rol Du Phyin Ma Yi Ge gChig Ma* (Skt. *Ekaksarimata-prajnaparamita*). She Rab sNa Tshogs, Kajur. Dege edition.

ZC: *bZang Po sPyod Pa'i sMon Lam Gyi rGyal Po* (Skt. *Bhadracharya-prani-dhana-raja*). Vol. Ah, Phal Bo Ch'e, Kajur. Dege edition.

ZN: *bDe Ba Chan Du sKye Ba 'Zhin Pa'i Ch'o Ga mDor bsDus Zhing mCh'og bGrod Pa'i Nye Lam,* by Jigme Tenpe Nyima.

Bibliography